Chondral Disease of the Knee

Chondral Disease of the Knee

A Case-Based Approach

Brian J. Cole, MD, MBA
Associate Professor, Department of Orthopedics
and Department of Anatomy and Cell Biology
Director, Cartilage Restoration Center at Rush
Rush University Medical Center, Chicago, Illinois

M. Mike Malek, MD
Director, Washington Orthopaedic and Knee Clinic, Fairfax, Virginia
President, National Knee Research and Education Foundation,
Clinton, Maryland

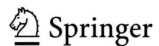 Springer

Brian J. Cole, MD, MBA
Associate Professor,
Department of Orthopedics and
  Department of Anatomy and
  Cell Biology; Director, Cartilage
  Restoration Center at Rush
Rush University Medical Center
Chicago, IL 60612
USA

M. Mike Malek, MD
Director, Washington Orthopaedic and
  Knee Clinic, Fairfax, VA 22031
President, National Knee Research
  and Education Foundation
  Clinton, MD 20735
USA

Library of Congress Control Number: 2005937074

ISBN 10: 0-387-30830-X
ISBN 13: 978-0387-30830-2

Printed in China. (BS/EVB)

9 8 7 6 5 4 3 2 1

springer.com

Contents

Contents

Section Editors

Brian J. Cole, MD, MBA
Department of Orthopedics
Department of Anatomy and Cell Biology
Cartilage Restoration Center at Rush
Rush University Medical Center
Chicago, IL 60612
USA

Michael G. Dennis, MD
Orthopaedic Care Center
Aventura Hospital and Medical Center
Aventura, FL 33180
USA

Contributors

Tim Bryant, RN
Brian J. Cole, MD, MBA
Jack Farr, MD
Tom Minas, MD, MS

Introduction to Case Studies

The illustrated case studies were prepared to help solidify the decision-making required for patients who are diagnosed with chondral disease of the knee. The cases are organized by level of complexity, taking into consideration substantial comorbidities such as tibiofemoral and patellofemoral malalignment, ligament disruption, and meniscal deficiency. The cases are presented in increasing level of difficulty based upon the defect- and patient-specific factors considered in the final treatment recommendation. Similar to the way a downhill ski run is graded for its level of difficulty, the cases are rated using green circles (easiest decision-making), blue squares (intermediate decision-making), black diamonds (advanced decision-making), and double black diamonds (expert decision-making). Within each category, the cases are organized by increasing complexity as well. Based upon the reader's practice experience, some may feel more comfortable with the decisions made in one category versus another. We believe, however, that this is the best way to convey the implicit level of complexity, thereby allowing the reader to better understand how these cases fall within the treatment algorithm. When off-label usage of technology was implemented, it is clearly indicated within the body of the case. While mastering the techniques and performing a thorough evaluation of all patient- and defect-specific factors is a prerequisite to sound judgment, the bullet points at the end of each case that emphasize the final rationale for the treatment chosen will be of particular interest and value to the reader.

Brian J. Cole, MD, MBA
M. Mike Malek, MD

Genzyme Biosurgery is proud to have collaborated with Springer to support the publication of this book. We are committed to improving patient care through education, research and advancing the field of cartilage repair. We applaud the efforts of the book's contributors and believe this text will be a valuable reference for clinicians seeking expert guidance in this emerging field.

Genzyme Biosurgery
A division of Genzyme Corporation
Cambridge, MA

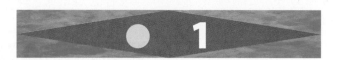

PATHOLOGY
Osteochondritis dissecans of the medial femoral condyle with documented long-term natural history

TREATMENT
Nonoperative treatment

SUBMITTED BY
Brian J. Cole, MD, MBA, Rush Cartilage Restoration Center, Rush University Medical Center, Chicago, Illinois, USA

CHIEF COMPLAINT AND HISTORY OF PRESENT ILLNESS

The patient is currently a 39-year-old male orthopedic surgeon who was diagnosed with symptomatic osteochondritis dissecans of his medial femoral condyle of his left knee at the age of 14. At that time, he complained of weight-bearing pain and discomfort on the medial aspect of his left knee with activity-related swelling. When initially diagnosed as having osteochondritis dissecans, he was treated with 8 weeks of nonweight bearing with crutches and asked to refrain from sports or impact activities thereafter. He remained asymptomatic, but was followed up regularly for radiographic evaluation to assess for evidence of instability.

PHYSICAL EXAMINATION

He ambulates with a nonantalgic gait and stands in symmetric physiologic varus. He has no effusion and full range of motion. He has no tenderness over his medial femoral condyle. His entire knee examination is normal.

RADIOGRAPHIC EVALUATION

A series of radiographs obtained from the age of 14 to the present demonstrate persistence of the osteochondritis dissecans lesion with no progression or evidence of instability. Radiographs demonstrate a lesion of osteochondritis dissecans of the medial femoral condyle of his left knee (Figures C1.1 through C1.3).

FOLLOW-UP

The patient remains completely asymptomatic and active in several high-level sports including skiing and running. Serial radiographs demonstrate persistence of the lesion.

DECISION-MAKING FACTORS

1. Diagnosed early at a time when growth plates remained open.
2. Initial attempt at nonoperative treatment with protected weight bearing was successful in rendering him asymptomatic.
3. Despite persistence of the lesion demonstrated on plain radiographs and magnetic resonance imaging (MRI), he remains asymptomatic and highly active.
4. An identified target lesion that can be reliably followed clinically and radiographically for evidence of progression or instability.

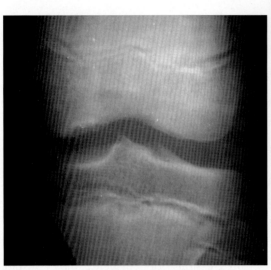

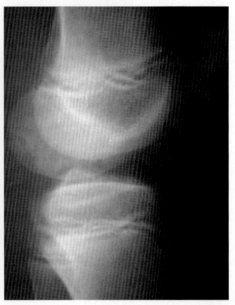

A

B

FIGURE C1.1. Initial radiographs of a 14-year-old male with symptomatic osteochondritis dissecans of the left knee. Anteroposterior (A) and lateral (B) radiographs demonstrate an in situ lesion of osteochondritis dissecans of the medial femoral condyle.

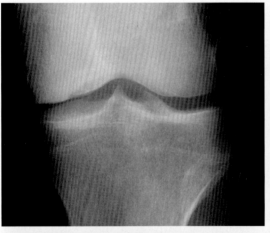

A

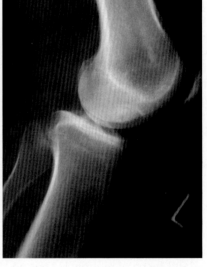

B

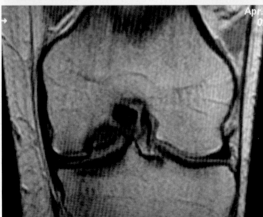

C

FIGURE C1.2. Radiographs obtained 24 years later. Anteroposterior (A) and lateral (B) radiographs demonstrate no evidence of fragmentation or collapse. (C) Coronal MRI demonstrates no fragmentation or evidence of significant instability.

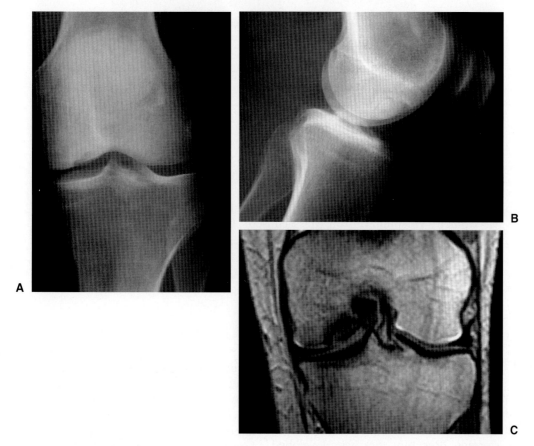

FIGURE C1.3. Radiographs obtained 29 years later. Anteroposterior **(A)** and lateral **(B)** radiographs demonstrate no evidence of fragmentation or collapse. **(C)** Coronal MRI demonstrates no fragmentation or evidence of significant instability. No significant interval change is seen compared to Figure C1.2.

PATHOLOGY
Avascular necrosis

PROCEDURE
Total knee replacement

SUBMITTED BY
Tom Minas, MD, and Tim Bryant, RN, Cartilage Repair Center, Brigham and Women's Hospital, Boston, Massachusetts, USA

CHIEF COMPLAINT AND HISTORY OF PRESENT ILLNESS

The patient is a 55-year-old man with a long-standing history of ulcerative colitis. His acute episodes have been treated with high-dose steroids. Recently, he has developed severe right knee weight-bearing discomfort. He also has pain at rest and at night. The joint pain is confined to his right knee only. He denies generalized malaise, fever, or erythema of the knee joint. Antiinflammatory medications and corticosteroid injections have not helped. He is unable to walk without the use of a cane.

PHYSICAL EXAMINATION

Height, 5 ft, 11 in.; weight, 185 lb. Clinical examination demonstrates a severe antalgic gait without the use of a cane. He has a large joint effusion that limits his range of motion to 95 degrees of flexion. He has a 30-degree fixed flexion deformity. Tricompartmental crepitus is present with generalized tenderness. Ligament examination is unremarkable.

RADIOGRAPHIC EVALUATION

Plain radiographs demonstrate diffuse patchy osteopenia of the distal femur, patella, and proximal tibia with well-maintained joint spaces and some early flattening to the medial femoral condyle consistent with multifocal avascular necrosis (Figure C2.1). A magnetic resonance imaging (MRI) scan demonstrates diffuse distal femoral avascular necrosis (not shown), with an osteochondral fragment of the medial femoral condyle.

SURGICAL INTERVENTION

A cruciate-retaining total knee arthroplasty was performed (Figure C2.2). Aggressive physical therapy was required to restore full extension that was obtained at the time of surgery. A Dyasplint™ was utilized to assist in regaining extension and for stretching of the hamstrings and joint capsule.

FOLLOW-UP

Three months postoperatively, the patient regained 0 to 110 degrees of flexion. He walks with no gait disturbance and is painfree. Two years postoperatively his result remains excellent.

FIGURE C2.1. Standing anteroposterior radiograph demonstrates normal tibiofemoral joint space, osteochondral defect of medial femoral condyle, early peripheral lateral osteophytes, and patchy sclerosis and lucency of the distal femur compatible with avascular necrosis.

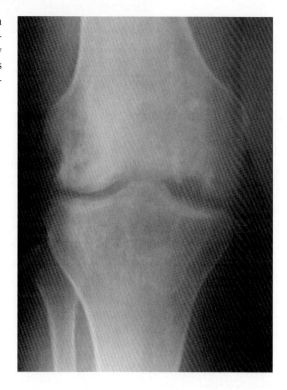

DECISION-MAKING FACTORS

1. Low-demand, 55-year-old male with severely symptomatic multifocal avascular necrosis.

2. Ongoing use of oral steroids.
3. Global nature of avascular necrosis and ongoing steroid insult contraindicates the implementation of cartilage restoration.

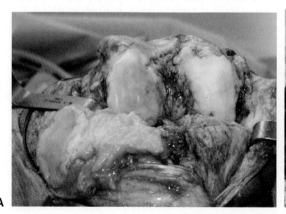
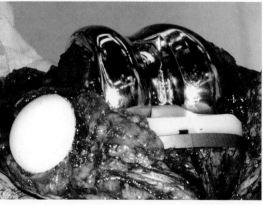

A   B

FIGURE C2.2. **(A)** Clinical photograph at the time of arthrotomy reveals discolored articular cartilage that is easily peeled off the distal femur. **(B)** Intraoperative appearance of total knee prosthesis.

PATHOLOGY
Unstable in situ osteochondritis dissecans of the medial femoral condyle

TREATMENT
Arthroscopic fixation of osteochondral fragment followed by hardware removal

SUBMITTED BY
Brian J. Cole, MD, MBA, Rush Cartilage Restoration Center, Rush University Medical Center, Chicago, Illinois, USA

CHIEF COMPLAINT AND HISTORY OF PRESENT ILLNESS

The patient is a 14-year-old girl with a 1-year history of weight-bearing pain and discomfort on the medial aspect of her right knee with activity-related swelling and mechanical symptoms. When initially diagnosed as having osteochondritis dissecans, she was treated with 8 weeks of nonweight bearing with crutches and asked to refrain from sports or impact activities thereafter. Despite these efforts, she remained symptomatic and was referred for definitive treatment.

PHYSICAL EXAMINATION

Height, 5ft, 3in.; weight, 115lb. She ambulates with a slightly antalgic gait and stands in symmetric physiologic valgus. Her right knee has a moderate-sized effusion. Her range of motion is 0 to 130 degrees. She is tender to palpation over the medial femoral condyle. Meniscal findings are absent. Her patellofemoral joint demonstrates normal tracking with no evidence of crepitus or apprehension. Her ligament examination is within normal limits.

RADIOGRAPHIC EVALUATION

Radiographs demonstrate an unstable lesion of osteochondritis dissecans of the medial femoral condyle of her right knee (Figure C3.1).

SURGICAL INTERVENTION

Because of persistent symptoms, she was indicated for arthroscopic reduction and internal fixation using a headless titanium screw. At arthroscopy, a lesion approximately 20mm by 20mm was found to be in situ, but unstable, with two palpably loose fragments. The fragments were elevated from the bed while leaving it hinged on an intact portion of the articular cartilage, and the base was debrided and microfractured. The fragments were repaired with two titanium headless screws (Acutrak, Mansfield, MA, USA) (Figure C3.2). Postoperatively, the patient was made nonweight bearing for approximately 8 weeks and utilized a continuous passive motion machine. At 8 weeks, she returned for hardware removal whereby the defect was believed to be stable and fully healed (Figures C3.3, C3.4). She was permitted to return to all activities at 4 months following her hardware removal.

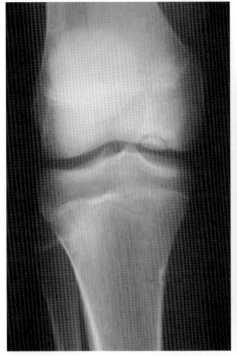
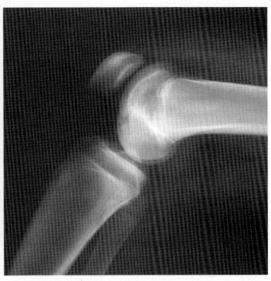

A   **B**

FIGURE C3.1. Anteroposterior **(A)** and lateral **(B)** radiographs demonstrate in situ lesion of osteochondritis dissecans of the medial femoral condyle in the right knee of a skeletally immature adolescent. Note the fragmentation best seen on the lateral radiograph.

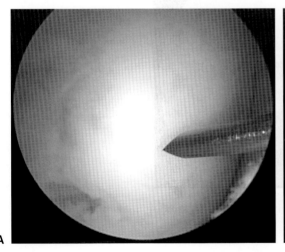
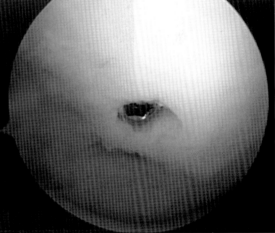

A   **B**

FIGURE C3.2. **(A)** An unstable lesion of osteochondritis dissecans seen arthroscopically along the medial femoral condyle. **(B)** The lesion bed has been prepared with debridement and microfracture followed by arthroscopic fixation using headless titanium screws for compression.

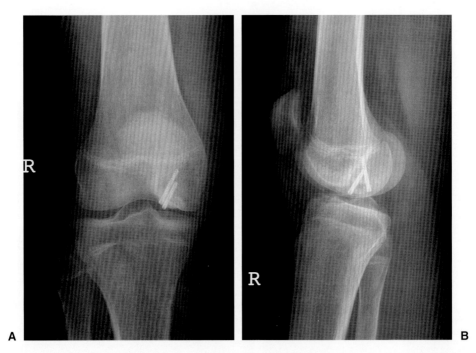

FIGURE C3.3. Anteroposterior **(A)** and lateral **(B)** radiographs obtained 8 weeks postoperatively demon-strate excellent healing of the fragment with no evidence of displacement.

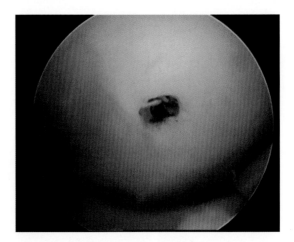

FIGURE C3.4. Eight-week arthroscopic view immediately following screw removal demonstrates clinical evi-dence of union of the osteochondral fragment.

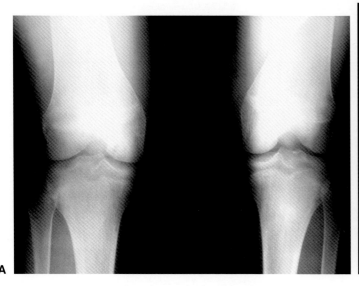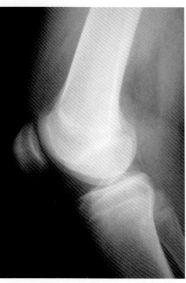

A   B

FIGURE C3.5 Six-month postoperative anteroposterior **(A)** and lateral **(B)** radiographs demonstrate integration of the fragment with no evidence of further fragmentation.

FOLLOW-UP

At the patient's 6-month follow-up visit, she had no symptoms and had returned to all activities. Radiographs demonstrate a healed osteochondritis dissecans lesion of the medial femoral condyle (Figure C3.5).

DECISION-MAKING FACTORS

1. Young patient with symptomatic lesion of osteochondritis dissecans.

2. Persistent symptoms despite initial treatment with nonoperative protocol.
3. In situ, but unstable, lesion without significant fragmentation and clinically viable osteochondral fragment large enough to be repaired with screws.
4. Despite need for hardware removal, compression fixation used to maximize chances for healing.

PATHOLOGY

Unstable in situ osteochondritis dissecans of the medial femoral condyle

TREATMENT

Arthroscopic fixation of osteochondral fragment followed by loose body removal

SUBMITTED BY

Brian J. Cole, MD, MBA, Rush Cartilage Restoration Center, Rush University Medical Center, Chicago, Illinois, USA

CHIEF COMPLAINT AND HISTORY OF PRESENT ILLNESS

The patient is an active 35-year-old woman who had no previous history of knee problems until the insidious onset of medial-sided right knee pain, swelling, and weight-bearing discomfort that began 6 months before presentation. She denied any trauma and was actively participating in snow skiing, running, and aerobics before the onset of these symptoms. She does not ever recall knee symptoms as a child or adolescent. She was referred for treatment of an unstable lesion of osteochondritis dissecans (OCD).

PHYSICAL EXAMINATION

Height, 5 ft, 5 in.; weight, 135 lb. She ambulates with a nonantalgic gate. She stands in symmetric physiologic valgus. Her right knee has a moderate-sized effusion. Her range of motion is 0 to 130 degrees. She is tender to palpation over the medial femoral condyle and has crepitus along the medial side of her knee with range of motion. Meniscal findings are absent. Her ligament examination is within normal limits.

RADIOGRAPHIC EVALUATION

Preoperative radiographs demonstrate a fragmented lesion of OCD along the medial femoral condyle in the right knee (Figure C4.1).

SURGICAL INTERVENTION

Because of the nature of her symptoms and the radiographic findings, she was indicated for an initial attempt at arthroscopic reduction and fixation of the OCD lesion. At the time of arthroscopy, an unstable lesion measuring approximately 2 cm by 3 cm by 1 cm (depth) was found in situ. A single major fragment was appreciated with a smaller minor fragment. This entire lesion was elevated from its bed, and the base was debrided and microfractured to promote healing. The major fragment was reduced and repaired with a single headless titanium screw (Acutrak, Mansfield, MA). The minor fragment was too small for screw fixation, and a single bioabsorbable pin was used (Orthosorb Pin; Johnson and Johnson, Canton, MA) (Figure C4.2). Postoperatively, the patient was made nonweight bearing for approximately 8 weeks and utilized continuous passive motion at 6 h/day. Thereafter, she was allowed to gradually return to higher-level activities.

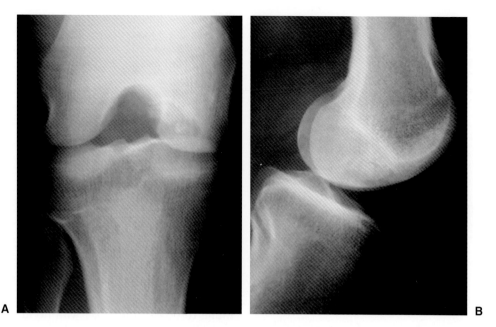

FIGURE C4.1. Preoperative anteroposterior **(A)** and lateral **(B)** radiographs demonstrate a fragmented lesion of osteochondritis dissecans (OCD) along the medial femoral condyle of the right knee.

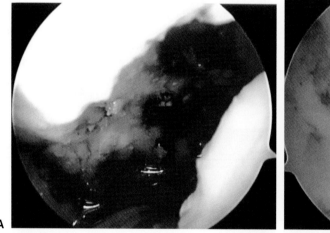
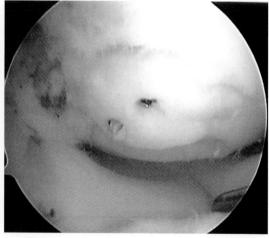

FIGURE C4.2. **(A)** An unstable lesion of OCD is seen arthroscopically along the medial femoral condyle with the lesion hinged open on intact articular cartilage. The base is debrided and microfractured to promote healing. **(B)** Arthroscopic fixation achieved with a headless titanium screw (Acutrak, Mansfield, MA) and a single bioabsorbable pin (Orthosorb Pin, Johnson and Johnson, Canton, MA).

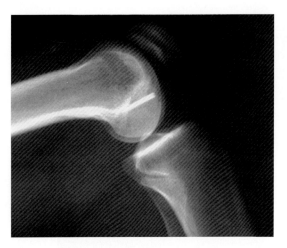

FIGURE C4.3. Lateral radiographs obtained at 1 year demonstrate a loose body within the suprapatellar pouch. Otherwise, the main fragment appears intact with the hardware still in place.

FOLLOW-UP

The patient did exceptionally well until she presented again 1 year later with complaints of mechanical locking. However, the weight-bearing pain along the medial aspect of her knee was completely eliminated. Postoperative radiographs taken at 1 year demonstrated a loose body within the suprapatellar pouch, seen best on the lateral radiograph (Figure C4.3). She was indicated for arthroscopy for removal of the loose body. The defect was inspected and found to be entirely intact with no identifiable source for the loose body, although it was suspected that the minor fragment had displaced and its bed had filled with fibrocartilage (Figure C4.4). The headless screw was deep within the subchondral bone and completely overgrown with fibrocartilage and was, therefore, not removed. The patient returned to all activities, and radiographs taken at 2 years postoperatively demonstrated no evidence of further

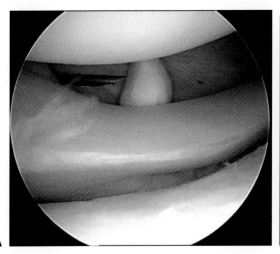

A

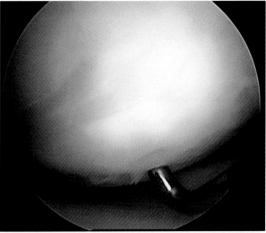

B

FIGURE C4.4. **(A)** Arthroscopic view of the loose body within the posterior aspect of the lateral compartment near the popliteal tendon. **(B)** Arthroscopic view of the defect without any obvious source of the loose body. The defect is stable to palpation and the areas are covered with fibrocartilage.

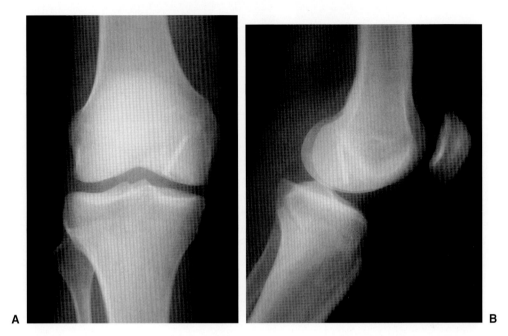

FIGURE C4.5 Two-year postoperative anteroposterior **(A)** and lateral **(B)** radiographs demonstrate osseous integration of the main fragment and no evidence of further fragmentation.

fragmentation with osseous integration of the major fragment (Figure C4.5).

DECISION-MAKING FACTORS

1. In situ defect with a viable plate of subchondral bone attached to the defect.

2. The ability to achieve anatomic fixation within the defect bed and a strong desire to avoid future treatment required for cartilage restoration should the fragment otherwise be removed.

3. Compression fixation used despite potential need for hardware removal to maximize chances for healing.

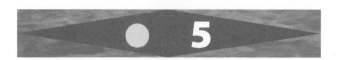

PATHOLOGY

Concomitant medial meniscus tear and focal chondral defect of the medial femoral condyle

TREATMENT

Medial meniscectomy and microfracture medial femoral condyle

SUBMITTED BY

Brian J. Cole, MD, MBA, Rush Cartilage Restoration Center, Rush University Medical Center, Chicago, Illinois, USA

CHIEF COMPLAINT AND HISTORY OF PRESENT ILLNESS

This 40-year-old woman had no preexisting knee problems until a twisting event occurred while attempting to squat. She noted the sudden onset of right knee pain and locking along the medial aspect of her knee. Her pain did not remit despite the passage of approximately 12 weeks time, and she continued to complain of locking. Because of her clinical symptoms, she was indicated for arthroscopy with a presumed diagnosis of medial meniscus tear.

PHYSICAL EXAMINATION

Height, 5 ft, 4 in.; weight, 130 lb. She ambulated with a slight antalgic gait. She stood in slight symmetric physiologic valgus. Her right knee has a small effusion. She is tender to palpation over the medial joint line. She has a positive flexion McMurray's test. Her range of motion is 0 to 120 degrees, with pain upon further attempt at flexion. Ligamentous testing is within normal limits.

RADIOGRAPHIC EVALUATION

Plain radiographs were within normal limits. No magnetic resonance image (MRI) was obtained.

SURGICAL INTERVENTION

At the time of the arthroscopy, she was noted to have a posterior horn medial meniscus tear with an irreparable parrot-beak configuration. The patient underwent a partial arthroscopic meniscectomy with debridement to a stable rim (Figure C5.1). Additionally, an incidental grade IV chondral lesion of the medial femoral condyle measuring approximately 15 mm by 15 mm was noted, which was questionably contributing to her symptoms. In part because the lesion was present in the ipsilateral symptomatic compartment, a formal microfracture technique was performed (Figure C5.2). Postoperatively, the patient was made nonweight bearing for 6 weeks and placed on continuous passive motion. There-

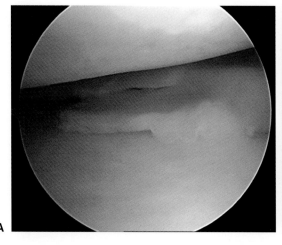
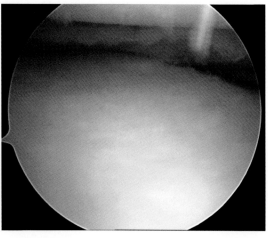

A   B

FIGURE C5.1. Arthroscopic photographs demonstrating an irreparable, parrot-beak configuration tear of the posterior horn of the medial meniscus before **(A)** and after **(B)** partial meniscectomy back to a stable rim.

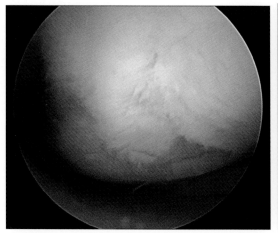
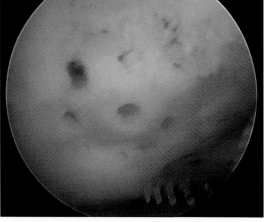

A   B

FIGURE C5.2. Photographs of grade III/IV chondral lesion of the medial femoral condyle measuring approximately 15 mm by 15 mm before **(A)** and after **(B)** formal microfracture technique was performed.

after, she gradually progressed to activities as tolerated.

FOLLOW-UP

At 2 years of follow-up, she has continued to do well with the absence of any activity-related effusions, swelling, or ongoing discomfort.

DECISION-MAKING FACTORS

1. Simple irreparable meniscus tear that should predictably respond favorably to meniscectomy.
2. An incidental chondral lesion of the medial femoral condyle that could or might be a cause of persistent symptoms if left untreated.

3. A chondral lesion of relatively small size (i.e., less than 2–3 cm^2) in an otherwise low activity level and low physical demand patient.

4. Anticipated willingness of the patient to comply with the early-phase rehabilitation requirements to optimize the results following a marrow-stimulating technique.

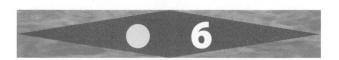

> **PATHOLOGY**
> Isolated focal chondral defect of the medial femoral condyle
>
> **TREATMENT**
> Microfracture
>
> **SUBMITTED BY**
> Tom Minas, MD and Tim Bryant, RN, Cartilage Repair Center, Brigham and
> Women's Hospital, Boston, Massachusetts, USA

CHIEF COMPLAINT AND HISTORY OF PRESENT ILLNESS

The patient is a 48-year-old woman who sustained an injury to the medial femoral condyle of her right knee. This lesion was treated with arthroscopic debridement alone for a grade II, partial-thickness chondral defect. This intervention alleviated her catching symptoms; however, her medial-sided weight-bearing pain persisted. She had significant limitations of her activities of daily living. She was not a particularly athletic or active individual, but desired pain relief with activities of daily living.

PHYSICAL EXAMINATION

Height, 5 ft, 3 in.; weight, 125 lb. Clinical examination demonstrated a slim woman with neutrally aligned lower extremities. She had no gait disturbance. Her range of motion was full and symmetric. There was no effusion. She had tenderness over the weight-bearing portion of her medial femoral condyle. Her ligament and meniscal examinations were normal.

RADIOGRAPHIC EVALUATION

Plain films were unremarkable and were without evidence of joint space narrowing or degenerative changes.

SURGICAL INTERVENTION

At arthroscopy, a small 10 mm by 10 mm grade III lesion of the medial femoral condyle was identified. A formal microfracture technique was performed, including removal and curettage of damaged repair tissue and cartilage back to stable intact normal articular cartilage; this involved removal of the tidemark. A sharp microfracture awl was used peripherally around the defect and then centrally at intervals of 3 to 5 mm without connecting or destabilizing the subchondral plate (Figure C6.1). Postoperatively, the patient was made protected weight bearing for 6 weeks and used continuous passive motion.

FOLLOW-UP

The patient was full weight bearing by 3 months and returned to sporting activities by 6 months. She is presently 1 year after her surgery and is pain-free (Figure C6.2).

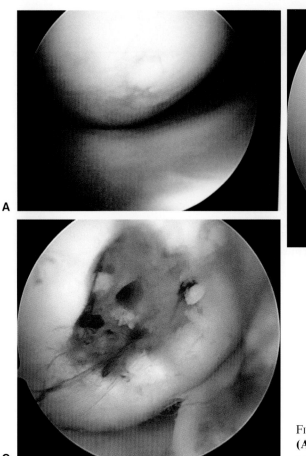

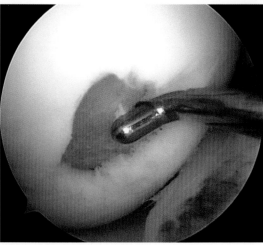

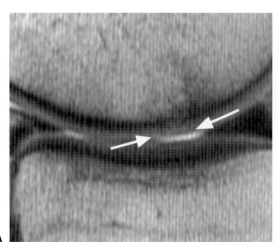

FIGURE C6.1. Arthroscopic photographs identifying **(A)** 10 mm by 10 mm defect treated with **(B)** defect preparation and **(C)** microfracture technique.

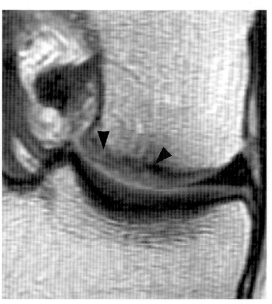

FIGURE C6.2. One-year postoperative magnetic resonance imaging (MRI) demonstrates on sagittal **(A)** and coronal **(B)** images that repair tissue is filling the defect area, where former microfracture was performed (*arrows*).

DECISION-MAKING FACTORS

1. Low-demand patient with small focal chondral defect which represented a relatively large area of the entire width of the medial femoral condyle.
2. Failure of previous arthroscopic debridement.
3. Osteochondral autograft was not chosen due to concerns for donor site morbidity given relatively small size of the trochlea.
4. Willingness to remain compliant with post-operative rehabilitation required to achieve successful result following microfracture.
5. Patient understanding that excessive activity levels, despite fibrocartilage fill, may lead to recurrent symptoms and further treatment attempts.

PATHOLOGY

Symptomatic focal chondral defect of lateral femoral condyle

TREATMENT

Microfracture of lateral femoral condyle with biopsy for possible future autologous chondrocyte implantation

SUBMITTED BY

Brian J. Cole, MD, MBA, Rush Cartilage Restoration Center, Rush University Medical Center, Chicago, Illinois, USA

CHIEF COMPLAINT AND HISTORY OF PRESENT ILLNESS

This patient is a 39-year-old, very active architect who had a hyperextension injury to his left knee while playing basketball. He had immediate onset of swelling and weight-bearing pain along the lateral aspect of his left knee. He failed to respond to conservative care. Because of his persistent symptoms that remained unresponsive to relative rest, a magnetic resonance image (MRI) was obtained; based upon this information, he was indicated for arthroscopy.

PHYSICAL EXAMINATION

Height, 5 ft, 10 in.; weight, 180 lb. The patient ambulates with a slightly antalgic gait. He stands in symmetric neutral alignment. His left knee has a moderate-sized effusion. His range of motion is from 0 to 130 degrees. He is tender to palpation over the lateral femoral condyle. Meniscal findings are absent. Patellofemoral joint demonstrates good tracking with no evidence of crepitus. His ligamentous examination is within normal limits.

RADIOGRAPHIC EVALUATION

Plain radiographs were evaluated and found to be within normal limits (Figure C7.1). MRI showed subchondral edema and violation of the chondral surface of the lateral femoral condyle (Figure C7.2).

SURGICAL INTERVENTION

At the time of arthroscopy, a full-thickness 10 mm by 16 mm chondral injury of the lateral femoral condyle within the weight-bearing zone in extension was identified (Figure C7.3). A formal microfracture procedure was performed (Figure C7.4). Because of the patient's relatively active lifestyle, the location of the lesion, and the possibility for fibrocartilage breakdown in the future, a concomitant biopsy of 200 to 300 mg cartilaginous tissue was obtained from the intercondylar notch (Figure C7.5). [The author of this case (B.J.C.) currently does not routinely biopsy a patient unless there is an explicit intention to treat a defect with autologous chondrocyte implantation in the near future.] Postoperatively, the patient was made non-weight bearing for approximately 6 weeks. He was placed on continuous passive motion, which he performed for 6 weeks at 6 h/day.

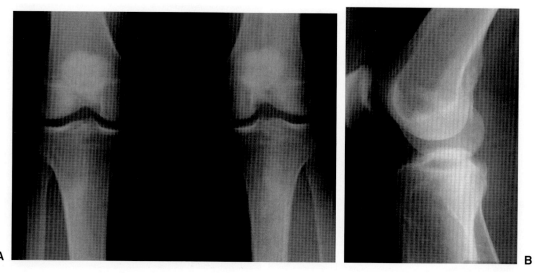

FIGURE C7.1. Forty-five-degree flexion weight-bearing posteroanterior (**A**) and lateral (**B**) radiographs demonstrate no abnormalities.

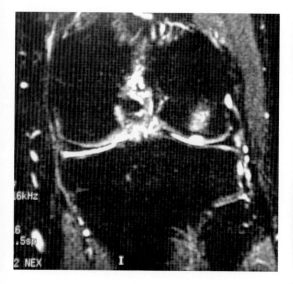

FIGURE C7.2. Coronal MRI demonstrates subchondral edema as well as violation of the chondral surface of the lateral femoral condyle.

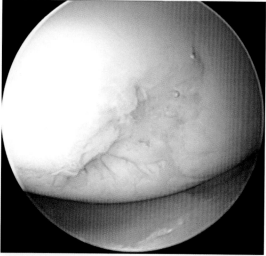

FIGURE C7.3. Arthroscopic photograph reveals a 10 mm by 16 mm full-thickness chondral dect of the lateral femoral condyle within the weight-bearing zone.

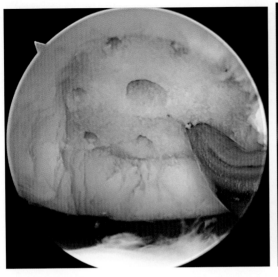
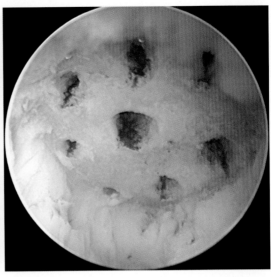

A

B

FIGURE C7.4. Arthroscopic views of the microfracture technique being performed. **(A)** Bloody return is shown from the holes penetrating the subchondral bone **(B)**.

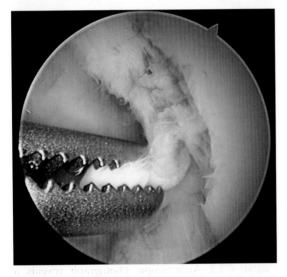

FIGURE C7.5. Arthroscopic view of biopsy of 200 to 300 mg cartilaginous tissue obtained from the intercondylar notch for potential future autologous chondrocyte implantation should the need arise.

FOLLOW-UP

The patient continues to do well nearly 2 years after his microfracture and has returned to all sports without any symptoms of weight-bearing pain, activity-related swelling, or discomfort. There is no intention in the near future to perform any further management of his defect unless he were to become symptomatic again.

DECISION-MAKING FACTORS

1. Relatively young active male with acute onset of symptoms related to a symptomatic femoral condyle chondral lesion.
2. Microfracture indicated as a first-time treatment for a relatively small chondral defect. Alternative treatment could also include primary osteochondral autograft transplantation.
3. Potential for failure of a marrow-stimulating technique in an otherwise active male, leading to the concomitant biopsy during this procedure.
4. Ability and willingness to be compliant with the postoperative rehabilitation required of a microfracture technique.

CHIEF COMPLAINT AND HISTORY OF PRESENT ILLNESS

This patient is a 31-year-old man who sustained a single, giving-way episode of his left knee, after a misstep approximately 4 months before evaluation. Since his initial injury, he has had several hyperextension-type giving-way episodes. He complains of activity-related swelling and medial knee pain with weight bearing. He is unable to participate in any impact-type activities.

PHYSICAL EXAMINATION

Height, 6 ft, 2 in.; weight, 188 lb. He ambulates with a nonantalgic gait. He stands in neutral alignment. His left knee has a moderate effusion. His range of motion is 0 to 130 degrees. He is tender to palpation over the medial femoral condyle. Meniscal findings are absent. His ligament examination is within normal limits.

RADIOGRAPHIC EVALUATION

Plain radiographs and magnetic resonance imaging (MRI) are within normal limits.

SURGICAL INTERVENTION

Because of his persistent symptoms, he was indicated for a diagnostic arthroscopy and evaluation for possible chondral injury. At the time of arthroscopy, he was noted to have a 10 mm by 10 mm grade IV lesion along the weight-bearing portion of his medial femoral condyle (Figure C8.1). It was elected to proceed with primary osteochondral autograft transplantation (Figure C8.2). Postoperatively, the patient

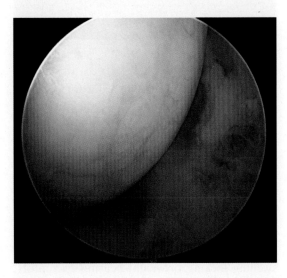

FIGURE C8.1. Arthroscopic photograph of the 10 mm by 10 mm lesion along the weight-bearing portion of his medial femoral condyle.

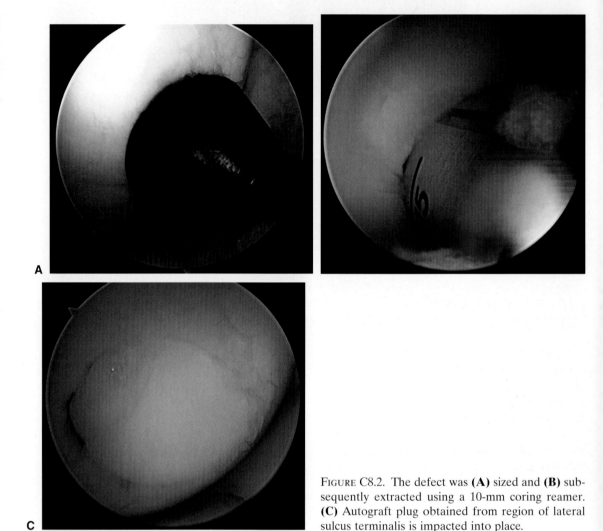

FIGURE C8.2. The defect was **(A)** sized and **(B)** subsequently extracted using a 10-mm coring reamer. **(C)** Autograft plug obtained from region of lateral sulcus terminalis is impacted into place.

was made partial weight bearing for approximately 4 to 6 weeks and placed on continuous passive motion for 6 weeks at approximately 6 h/day. Thereafter, he progressed to activities as tolerated.

FOLLOW-UP

At his 2-year follow-up, the patient complains of no pain. He has full range of motion and enjoys all sports without any symptoms such as swelling, locking, or weight-bearing discomfort.

DECISION-MAKING FACTORS

1. Defect less than 2cm^2 in the weight-bearing zone of the femoral condyle.
2. Isolated pathology in a young, active male with expectations and activity levels likely to exceed any benefit that microfracture might provide.
3. First-line treatment aimed at cartilage restoration because his activity level and the defect characteristics warranted this relatively higher level of treatment.

PATHOLOGY
Isolated medial compartment osteoarthritis

TREATMENT
Unicompartmental knee replacement

SUBMITTED BY
Tom Minas, MD, and Tim Bryant, RN, Cartilage Repair Center, Brigham and Women's Hospital, Boston, Massachusetts, USA

CHIEF COMPLAINT AND HISTORY OF PRESENT ILLNESS

The patient is a 60-year-old man with severe left knee medial joint line pain with weight bearing. He has difficulty walking even short distances. He also has difficulty with stairs. He has severe limitations with activities of daily living, and wishes to have pain relief with these activities as well as with nonimpact recreational sports. He has failed attempts at treatment with corticosteroid injections, unloader bracing, antiinflammatories, and physical therapy.

PHYSICAL EXAMINATION

Height, 5 ft, 11 in.; weight, 185 lb. The patient is a slender 60-year-old man who appears physiologically younger than his chronologic age. He has mild symmetric varus alignment of both lower extremities. He walks with an antalgic gait on the left side only. His range of motion is 0 to 125 degrees of flexion. He has medial joint line tenderness and medial tibiofemoral crepitus. There is no effusion and no patellofemoral or lateral compartment crepitus or tenderness.

There are palpable medial osteophytes, and his alignment corrects almost to neutral with a valgus-producing force. There is a good medial endpoint. His ligament examination is within normal limits.

RADIOGRAPHIC EVALUATION

Plain radiographs demonstrate complete loss of the medial joint space, and a healthy lateral and patellofemoral joint compartment without evidence of tibiofemoral subluxation (Figure C9.1).

SURGICAL INTERVENTION

Because of his age, low-demand activities, and need to return to work in a short period of time, it was decided to pursue surgical reconstruction by medial unicompartmental arthroplasty (Figure C9.2). Postoperatively, the patient was advanced to weight bearing and range of motion as tolerated. He progressed to activities as tolerated by 16 weeks (Figure C9.2).

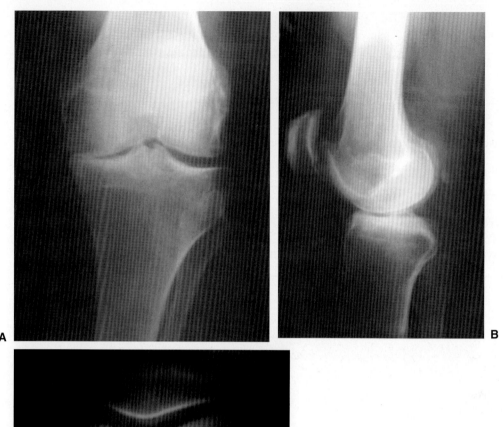

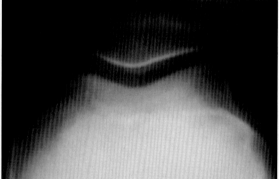

FIGURE C9.1. Preoperative **(A)** standing antero-posterior, **(B)** lateral, and **(C)** skyline radiographs demonstrate nearly complete loss of medial joint space with healthy lateral and patellofemoral compartments without evidence of tibiofemoral subluxation.

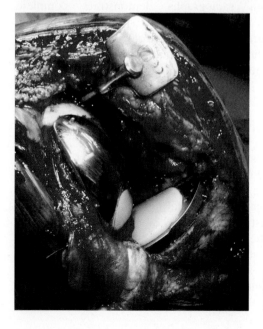

FIGURE C9.2. Intraoperative photograph of implanted tibiofemoral unicompartmental prosthesis through a minimally invasive incision without a quadriceps split.

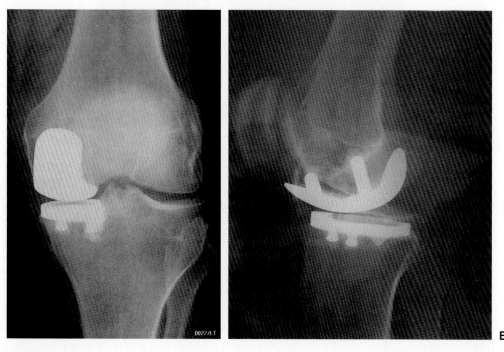

FIGURE C9.3. Postoperative anteroposterior **(A)** and lateral **(B)** radiographs of well-functioning medial uni-compartmental prosthesis.

FOLLOW-UP

Within a few weeks postoperatively his pain was completely resolved allowing early return to work. He returned to golf within 3 months and to recreational skiing within 9 months after reconstruction (Figure C9.3). His range of motion was comparable to his preoperative condition.

DECISION-MAKING FACTORS

1. An otherwise healthy, 60-year-old male with end-stage bipolar medial compartment osteoarthritis and slight varus alignment.
2. Goals: to return to low-demand activities and work within a few weeks of surgery.
3. No evidence of significant patellofemoral or lateral tibiofemoral symptoms by history, radiographs, or physical examination.

PATHOLOGY
Unicompartmental bipolar disease

TREATMENT
Unispacer

SUBMITTED BY
Jack Farr, MD, Cartilage Restoration Center of Indiana, OrthoIndy, Indianapolis, Indiana, USA.

CHIEF COMPLAINT AND HISTORY OF PRESENT ILLNESS

This male patient is a 44-year-old, large-machine mechanic with progressive, left greater than right, medial-sided knee pain. The quality is sharp with twisting and turning activities and at other times deep, dull aching. The severity is intense and the timing is per weight-bearing activity, although he does have some aching at rest. The patient has unsuccessfully worn an unloader knee brace for the past 2 years. He reports a history of an open meniscectomy and arthroscopy of his right knee performed more than 20 years previously. He smokes 1 to 2 packs per day and has for the past 20 years.

PHYSICAL EXAMINATION

Height, 5 ft, 9 in.; weight, 150 lb; BMI (body mass index), 22.5. The patient ambulates with an antalgic gait. He stands in slight symmetric varus. Bilateral range of motion is from 5 to 130 degrees of flexion. He has a mild effusion on the right knee and moderate effusion on the left knee. He has bilateral focal medial joint line tenderness. There is no increased ligamentous laxity.

RADIOGRAPHIC EVALUATION

Anteroposterior and lateral radiographs demonstrate medial compartment joint space narrowing (Figure C10.1). The Merchant view shows a central patella with maintenance of joint space. The posteroanterior standing notch view shows significant joint space loss in the right medial compartment and moderate narrowing in the left medial compartment. The long-leg alignment view shows 4 to 5 degrees varus on the right and 3 to 4 degrees varus on the left.

SURGICAL INTERVENTION

The arthroscopy revealed minimal chondrosis except medially where both the femoral condyle and tibial plateau had extensive grade III and early IV chondrosis. The meniscus was relatively absent. The anterior cruciate ligament was intact. Following arthroscopic preparation of the joint surfaces, a unispacer was inserted through a miniarthrotomy (Figure C10.2). Postoperatively, the patient was immediately allowed weight bearing and range of motion as tolerated. Advance to unrestricted activities was permitted after 3 months.

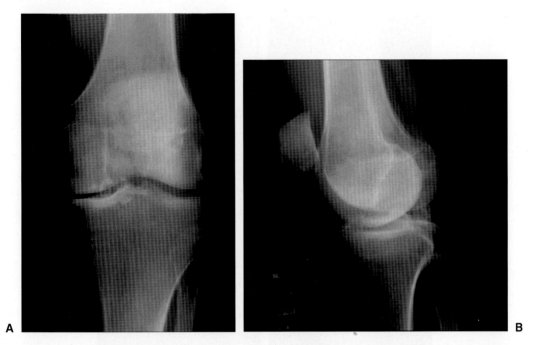

FIGURE C10.1. Preoperative anteroposterior **(A)** and lateral **(B)** radiographs show narrowing of medial joint space with slight varus deformity.

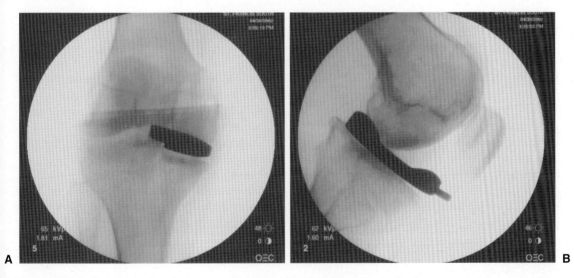

FIGURE C10.2. Intraoperative anteroposterior **(A)** and lateral **(B)** radiographs show proper placement of the unispacer.

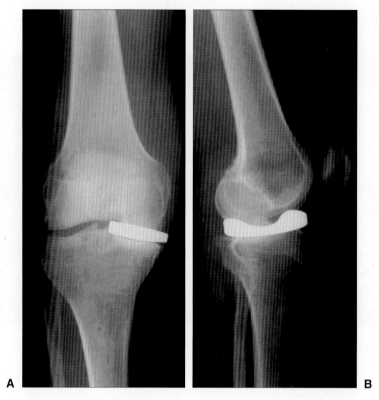

FIGURE C10.3. Three-month postoperative anteroposterior **(A)** and lateral **(B)** radiographs of unispacer in satisfactory position.

FOLLOW-UP

At 3 months, radiographs demonstrate good placement of the unispacer (Figure C10.3). The patient has returned to work and, at 6 months, he is now limited by his non-operative knee. He still has some minor complaints of residual discomfort along the medial side of his right knee, albeit less than he had preoperatively.

DECISION-MAKING FACTORS

1. Relatively advanced unicompartmental bipolar disease of the medial compartment in a young patient who is unwilling to take time off work to allow the healing required of a high tibial osteotomy.
2. A heavy smoker with a relative contraindication to osteotomy.
3. Considered to be relatively young for unicompartmental knee replacement.
4. Unispacer should allow successful revision, if necessary, to unicompartmental or total knee arthroplasty, without compromising the result of those procedures.

PATHOLOGY
Medial femoral condyle focal chondral defect

TREATMENT
Osteochondral autograft transplant

SUBMITTED BY
Brian J. Cole, MD, MBA, Rush Cartilage Restoration Center, Rush University Medical Center, Chicago, Illinois, USA

CHIEF COMPLAINT AND HISTORY OF PRESENT ILLNESS

This patient is a 42-year-old woman who had an acute twisting event and developed the onset of medial-sided right knee pain. She continued to complain of persistent right knee medial-sided weight-bearing pain and discomfort in addition to activity-related swelling. Her symptoms were not alleviated by a trial of antiinflammatory medication as well as a course of physical therapy.

PHYSICAL EXAMINATION

Height, 5 ft, 4 in.; weight, 155 lb. She has an antalgic gait. Her right knee has a moderate effusion. Her range of motion is 0 to 130 degrees. She is tender to palpation over the medial joint line and femoral condyle. Meniscal findings are equivocal, with pain reported with a varus axial load and rotation, but no palpable click. Her ligament examination is within normal limits.

RADIOGRAPHIC EVALUATION

Plain radiographs were unremarkable (Figure C11.1). A magnetic resonance image (MRI) was obtained and found to be within normal limits.

SURGICAL INTERVENTION

Initially, it was believed that she had a medial meniscus tear and was therefore indicated for arthroscopy. At arthroscopy, she was diagnosed as having an isolated grade III to IV chondral defect measuring 12 mm by 12 mm in the weight-bearing zone of the medial femoral condyle. As this was the only pathology identified, it was treated with an isolated microfracture technique (Figure C11.2). Postoperatively, the patient was made nonweight bearing for approximately 6 weeks and was placed on continuous passive motion for a similar period of time. She did well for approximately the first 8 months. As her activity level increased, however, she developed activity-related effusions and persistent medial-sided symptoms.

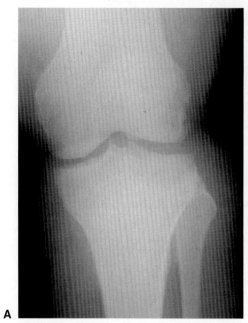
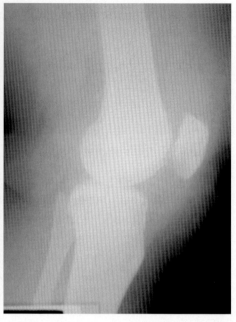

A   B

FIGURE C11.1. Anteroposterior **(A)** and lateral **(B)** radiographs of patient with a symptomatic medial femoral condyle chondral lesion diagnosed at arthroscopy, but with no evidence of defect demonstrated by plain radiographs or MRI.

Because of persistent symptoms, she was indicated for osteochondral autograft transplantation of the medial femoral condyle. At the time of surgery, there was significant fibro- cartilage fill of the medial femoral condyle, which was replaced with a 10-mm osteochondral autograft harvested from the lateral aspect of the trochlea (Figure C11.3).

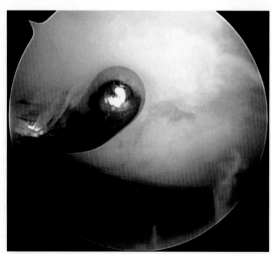
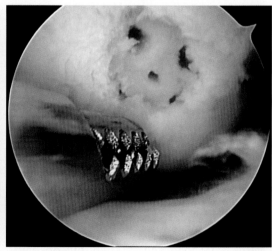

A   B

FIGURE C11.2. **(A)** Arthroscopic photograph of a grade III to grade IV lesion of the weight-bearing zone of the medial femoral condyle with delamination. **(B)** Microfracture technique used to treat this lesion.

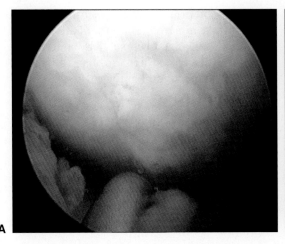
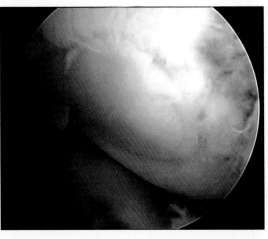

A   B

FIGURE C11.3. At second-look arthroscopy **(A)**, there is significant fibrocartilage fill within the previously microfractured defect. However, it is soft to palpation and the patient remains symptomatic. **(B)** Ten-millimeter osteochondral autograft plug impacted into place.

FOLLOW-UP

At 18 months postoperatively, the patient remains painfree and has resumed all her activities. Follow-up radiographs demonstrate excellent incorporation of the osteochondral autograft with no joint space narrowing, cystic change, or joint incongruity (Figure C11.4).

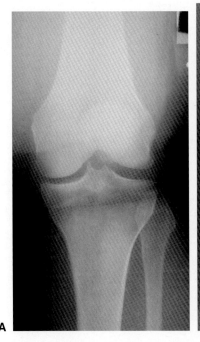
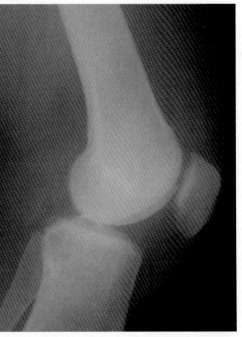

A   B

FIGURE C11.4. Anteroposterior **(A)** and lateral **(B)** radiographs, at 1-year follow-up demonstrate excellent incorporation of the osteochondral autograft without evidence of joint space narrowing, cystic change, or joint incongruity.

DECISION-MAKING FACTORS

1. Index microfracture in a symptomatic patient indicated for isolated lesion less than $2\,cm^2$ as a first-line treatment.

2. Failure of primary microfracture as index treatment in a young intermediate-demand patient with a relatively small isolated defect.

3. Ability to replace fibrocartilage fill with a single osteochondral autograft plug.

PATHOLOGY
Lateral femoral condyle focal chondral defect

TREATMENT
Osteochondral autograft transplant

SUBMITTED BY
Brian J. Cole, MD, MBA, Rush Cartilage Restoration Center, Rush University Medical Center, Chicago, Illinois, USA

CHIEF COMPLAINT AND HISTORY OF PRESENT ILLNESS

This patient is a 34-year-old emergency room nurse who sustained a work-related injury following a twisting event. She heard a pop and had the immediate onset of swelling and lateral-sided right knee pain. Subsequently, she reported a catching sensation but denied any episodes of giving-way. Her symptoms have not improved with a trial of antiinflammatory medication.

PHYSICAL EXAMINATION

Height, 5 ft, 4 in.; weight, 135 lb. She has a slightly antalgic gait with neutral alignment. Her right knee has a moderate-sized effusion. Her range of motion is 0 to 130 degrees. She is tender to palpation over the lateral femoral condyle. Meniscal findings are equivocal. Patellofemoral joint demonstrates good tracking with no evidence of crepitus. Her ligament examination is within normal limits.

RADIOGRAPHIC EVALUATION

Posteroanterior 45-degree flexion weight-bearing and lateral views were within normal limits (Figure C12.1). A magnetic resonance (MRI) was obtained that was significant for a suggestion of a type II signal within the lateral meniscus but was otherwise considered normal.

SURGICAL INTERVENTION

Because of failure to respond to conservative treatment, she was indicated for arthroscopic evaluation and treatment. At the time of arthroscopy, she was noted to have an isolated chondral lesion of the lateral femoral condyle measuring approximately 12 mm by 12 mm. This lesion was treated with a formal microfracture technique (Figure C12.2). Following the microfracture, the patient was placed non-weight bearing for approximately 4 to 6 weeks and used continuous passive motion for 4 to 6 h/day.

At the patient's 6-month follow-up visit, she continued to complain of persistent activity-related pain and swelling and was indicated for revision with an osteochondral autograft transplant. At arthroscopy, she had significant fibrocartilage fill of her previously microfractured defect (Figure C12.3). Osteochondral autograft transplantation was performed using 9-mm and 7-mm plugs obtained from the lateral trochlear ridge (Figure C12.4). Postoperatively, the patient was placed on protected weight bearing for approximately 4 to 6 weeks and uti-

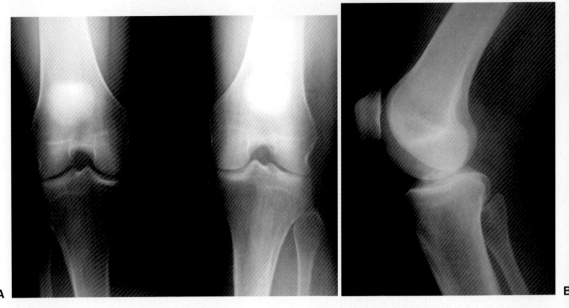

A   B

FIGURE C12.1. Forty-five-degree flexion posteroanterior weight-bearing **(A)** and lateral **(B)** radiographs without abnormalities.

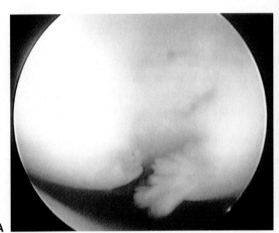

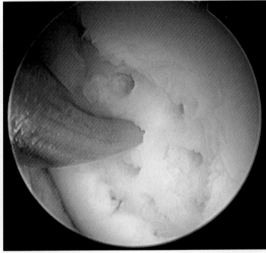

A   B

FIGURE C12.2. Index microfracture treatment of isolated 12 mm by 12 mm defect of the lateral femoral condyle. Arthroscopic view of the lesion **(A)** before microfracture and **(B)** after microfracture technique performed with creation of vertical walls surrounding the defect.

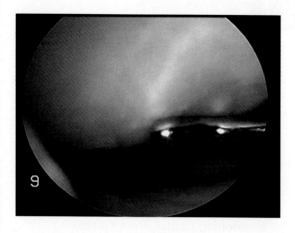

FIGURE C12.3. Arthroscopic view obtained 8 months after microfracture in which the defect was found to be filled with soft fibrocartilaginous tissue.

lized continuous passive motion. At 6 months, she was permitted to engage in activities as tolerated.

FOLLOW-UP

At nearly 1 year postoperatively, the patient has full range of motion, no swelling, and minimal complaints of activity-related pain.

DECISION-MAKING FACTORS

1. Index microfracture in a symptomatic patient indicated for isolated lesion less than 2 cm^2 as a first-line treatment.
2. Failure of primary microfracture as index treatment in a young intermediate-demand patient with a relatively small isolated defect.
3. Ability to replace fibrocartilage fill with two or fewer osteochondral autograft plugs.

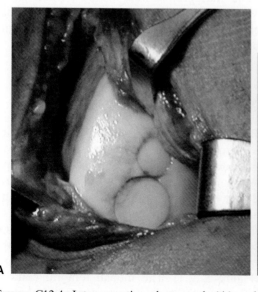
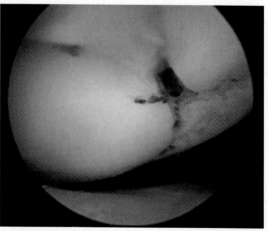

A   B

FIGURE C12.4. Intraoperative photograph **(A)** and arthroscopic view **(B)** of the osteochondral autograft transplant plugs, measuring 9 mm and 7 mm, respectively.

PATHOLOGY
Focal chondral defect of the medial femoral condyle and patella

TREATMENT
Osteochondral autograft of the medial femoral condyle and microfracture of the patella

SUBMITTED BY
Brian J. Cole, MD, MBA, Rush Cartilage Restoration Center, Rush University Medical Center, Chicago, Illinois, USA

CHIEF COMPLAINT AND HISTORY OF PRESENT ILLNESS

The patient is a 44-year-old woman with a chief complaint of anterior knee pain and pain with weight bearing along the medial aspect of her right knee. Additionally, she has recurrent mechanical symptoms, swelling, difficulty doing her work, and inability to participate in her hobby as a sport barrel jumper. Two years prior, she had an arthroscopic chondral debridement, and was diagnosed with a full-thickness chondral defect of her medial femoral condyle documented to be the "size of a dime" and a similarly sized, nearly full thickness lesion of her patella. She did not respond favorably to this arthroscopy and remained symptomatic. Before being indicated for repeat surgical intervention, she demonstrated a failure to respond to a rigorous patellofemoral rehabilitation program.

PHYSICAL EXAMINATION

Height, 5 ft, 4 in.; weight, 130 lb. The patient walks with a nonantalgic gait, and her alignment is symmetric in slight physiologic valgus. She has a small effusion. Her range of motion is 0 to 130 degrees. She is tender to palpation over the medial femoral condyle in flexion. She has palpable patellofemoral crepitus at 45 degrees of knee flexion with no patellar apprehension. Meniscal findings are absent, and her ligament examination is within normal limits. She has no quadriceps atrophy and has a Q angle of less than 8 degrees.

RADIOGRAPHIC EVALUATION

Plain radiographs were within normal limits. Magnetic resonance studies demonstrated both chondral lesions with subchondral edema behind the medial femoral condyle lesion.

SURGICAL INTERVENTION

Because of her persistent symptoms and failure to respond to previous debridement, she was indicated for a repeat right knee arthroscopy. An 8 mm by 8 mm, nearly grade IV chondral defect located centrally within the patella and an 8 mm by 8 mm, grade IV chondral defect of the weight-bearing zone of the medial femoral condyle were identified. The patellar lesion was treated with a formal microfracture technique (Figure C13.1). The medial femoral condyle lesion was treated with an osteochondral autograft transplant (Figure C13.2).

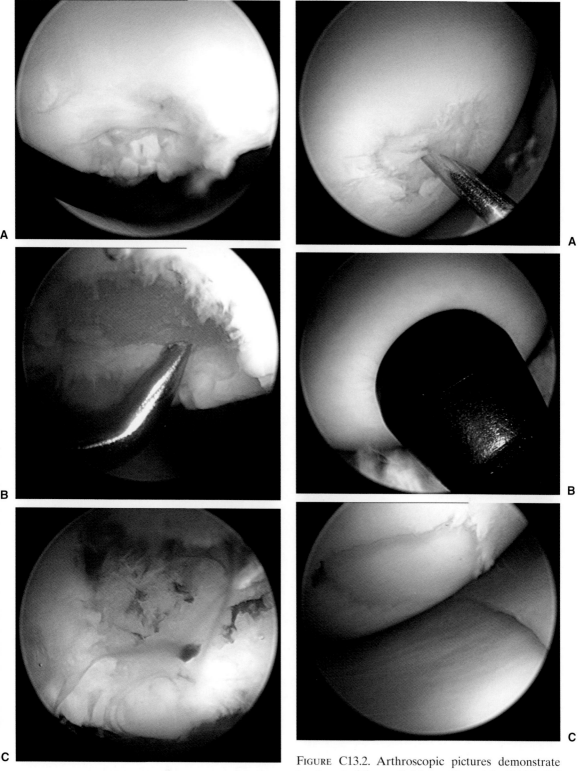

FIGURE C13.1. Arthroscopic pictures demonstrate treatment of patellar defect. **(A)** Central, nearly grade IV patellar defect measuring 8 mm by 8 mm. **(B)** Microfracture technique of the patella with debridement through the calcified layer and penetration with a microfracture awl. **(C)** Subchondral bone demonstrates bleeding through the microfracture holes.

FIGURE C13.2. Arthroscopic pictures demonstrate treatment of the medial femoral condyle. **(A)** Medial femoral condyle defect of the weight-bearing zone **(B)** being measured at approximately 8 mm by 8 mm. **(C)** The osteochondral plug in place.

FOLLOW-UP

In an effort to clear her for competitive barrel jumping and because she had mild anterior knee pain, the patient was indicated for second-look arthroscopy 6 months following her treatment. The patella demonstrated excellent fill with relatively soft fibrocartilaginous tissue, and the osteochondral plug demonstrated excellent integration with no evidence of degeneration (Figure C13.3). At 1 year, she reported only

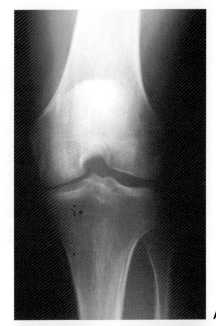

A

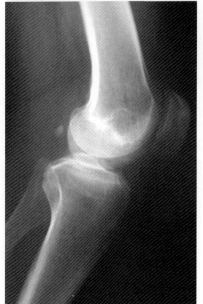

B

FIGURE C13.4. Two-year anteroposterior **(A)** and lateral **(B)** radiographs demonstrate virtually no evidence of the osteochondral plug and the absence of subchondral sclerosis or joint space narrowing.

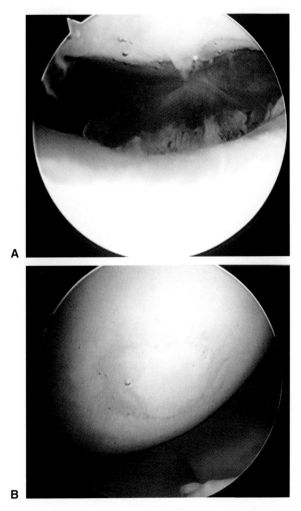

A

B

FIGURE C13.3. Six-month second-look arthroscopy of the patella **(A)** demonstrates soft fibrocartilage within the defect and the medial femoral condyle **(B)**, with a well-healed and integrated osteochondral autograft plug without signs of degeneration.

minimal activity-related symptoms, and at 2 years she was successfully competing at barrel jumping with no radiographic abnormalities (Figure C13.4).

DECISION-MAKING FACTORS

1. Physically demanding patient in her fifth decade with chondral lesions that failed to respond to initial arthroscopic debridement and physical therapy.
2. Small patellar lesion amenable to microfracture with few other viable or appropriate solutions. Other options considered could include anteromedialization osteotomy, depending on the severity of her symptoms.
3. Small lesion of the medial femoral condyle easily treated with a second-line treatment using a single-plug osteochondral autograft.

PATHOLOGY
Lateral femoral condyle osteochondritis dissecans

TREATMENT
Fresh osteochondral allograft transplantation

SUBMITTED BY
Brian J. Cole, MD, MBA, Rush Cartilage Restoration Center, Rush University Medical Center, Chicago, Illinois, USA

CHIEF COMPLAINT AND HISTORY OF PRESENT ILLNESS

This patient is a 19-year-old male college student whose chief complaint is that of activity-related lateral-sided left knee pain, with associated swelling, stiffness, locking, and a sense of giving-way. His symptom onset began suddenly 2 years previously while playing soccer. His symptoms are made worse with weight bearing, running, impact activities, and prolonged standing. He desires to participate in collegiate-level sports.

He was initially treated 1 year previously with arthroscopy and removal of a necrotic 2.5 cm by 2.5 cm osteochondral fragment consistent with chronic osteochondritis dissecans of the lateral femoral condyle (Figure C14.1). He failed to improve following loose body removal and was referred for definitive treatment.

PHYSICAL EXAMINATION

Height, 6 ft, 2 in.; weight, 185 lb. He has a normal gait. Alignment reveals slight symmetric physiologic varus of approximately 2 degrees. He has a mild effusion with tenderness along the lateral femoral condyle. His range of motion is from 0 to 130 degrees. There is no evidence of any meniscal findings. He has slight patellofemoral and lateral compartment crepitus with range of motion. He has no evidence of quadriceps atrophy. He has a normal patellofemoral joint and a normal ligament examination.

RADIOGRAPHIC EVALUATION

Forty-five-degree posteroanterior flexion weight-bearing and lateral radiographs demonstrate osteochondritis dissecans of the lateral femoral condyle of the left knee with a large cavitary defect involving more than 5 to 8 mm of subchondral bone at the base of the defect (Figure C14.2).

SURGICAL INTERVENTION

Because of the size, location, and depth of the lesion, the patient was indicated for fresh osteochondral allograft transplantation (Figure C14.3). Postoperatively, he was made non-weight bearing for approximately 8 weeks and used continuous passive motion for 6 weeks for 6 to 8 h/day. At 6 months, he was permitted to engage in high-impact activities.

FOLLOW-UP

Two years following his allograft transplant, he complains of no pain, swelling, or catching. He has returned to all activities. He has radiographic evidence of graft incorporation and preservation of joint space (Figure C14.4).

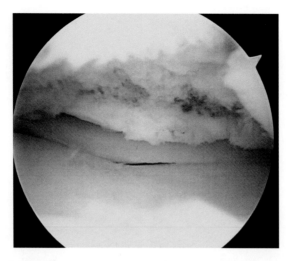

FIGURE C14.1. Arthroscopic photograph of the defect obtained at the time of fragment removal demonstrates exposed subchondral bone with normal meniscus and normal lateral tibial plateau.

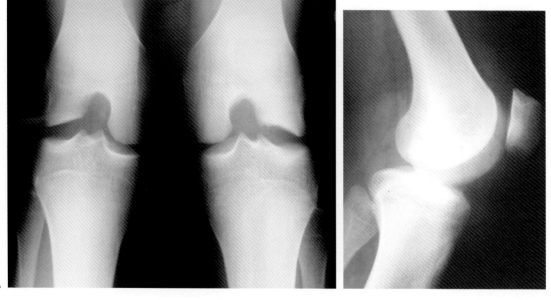

FIGURE C14.2. Forty-five-degree flexion posteroanterior weight-bearing **(A)** and lateral **(B)** radiographs demonstrate osteochondritis dissecans of the lateral femoral condyle of the left knee with a large cavitary defect.

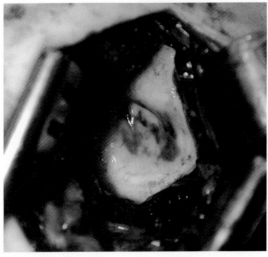
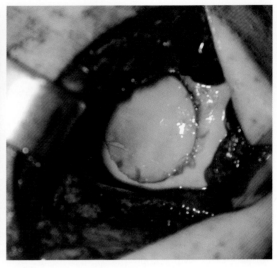

A

B

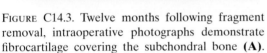

FIGURE C14.3. Twelve months following fragment removal, intraoperative photographs demonstrate fibrocartilage covering the subchondral bone **(A)**.

(B) Fresh osteochondral allograft, measuring 25 mm by 25 mm, is press-fit within the lateral femoral condyle.

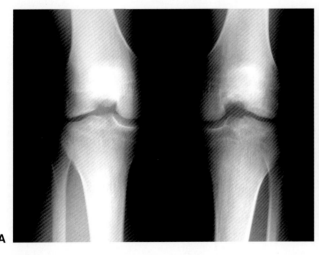
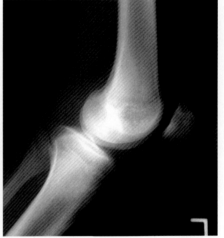

A

B

FIGURE C14.4. Two-year postoperative 45-degree flexion posteroanterior weight-bearing **(A)** and non-weight-bearing **(B)** flexion lateral radiographs

demonstrate excellent incorporation of the lateral femoral condyle osteochondral allograft.

DECISION-MAKING FACTORS

1. A young high-demand patient with osteochondritis dissecans of the weight-bearing
   zone of the lateral femoral condyle.
2. Failure of previous treatment involving fragment removal with persistent symptoms.
3. A large (6.25 cm²) and deep lesion (greater
   than 6 to 8 mm of subchondral bone involvement) of the lateral femoral condyle considered otherwise difficult if not contraindicated
   to manage with osteochondral autograft or
   autologous chondrocyte implantation.
4. Rehabilitation tolerance and willingness to
   be compliant with initial nonweight-bearing
   status.

PATHOLOGY
Focal chondral defect of the lateral femoral condyle

TREATMENT
Autologous chondrocyte implantation of the lateral femoral condyle

SUBMITTED BY
Brian J. Cole, MD, MBA, Rush Cartilage Restoration Center, Rush University Medical Center, Chicago, Illinois, USA

CHIEF COMPLAINT AND HISTORY OF PRESENT ILLNESS

The patient is a 27-year-old woman with a long-standing history of right knee patellar instability. As a child, before she was skeletally mature, she underwent two lateral releases that failed to resolve her instability. Subsequently, when she had reached skeletal maturity, she underwent an anteromedialization of her tibial tubercle. Although her patellar instability was successfully treated, she developed locking and mechanical symptoms requiring arthroscopic removal of several loose bodies approximately 2 years before presentation for cartilage treatment. At the time of the arthroscopy, she was noted to have an approximately 3 cm by 3 cm grade IV lesion in the lateral femoral condyle. She experienced some relief from the removal of the loose bodies; however, she still reports significant lateral-sided knee pain, swelling, and giving-way. Repeated attempts at formal physical therapy failed to alleviate her symptoms.

PHYSICAL EXAMINATION

Height, 5 ft, 3 in.; weight, 125 lb. She has a nonantalgic gait. She stands in slight symmetric physiologic valgus. She has a large lateral incision extending down inferiorly from her anteromedialization procedure and previous lateral releases. She has a trace effusion with mild patellofemoral crepitus. Her range of motion is from 0 to 135 degrees. She has a positive J sign with active extension. She has mild patellar apprehension with lateral glide testing in 30 degrees of flexion. She has significant tenderness over the lateral femoral condyle. Her medial and lateral joint lines are not tender. Her ligament exam is within normal limits.

RADIOGRAPHIC EVALUATION

Plain radiographs of the right knee (Figure C15.1) reveal hardware fixation from the previous anteromedialization procedure in place as well as an incongruity on the lateral femoral condyle of her left knee. Magnetic resonance imaging (MRI) examination reveals a chondral defect of the lateral femoral condyle with a full-thickness lesion extending into the subchondral bone with subchondral edema present.

SURGICAL INTERVENTION

The patient underwent arthroscopy in which a lateral femoral condyle defect with soft fibrocartilaginous tissue measuring 20 mm by 25 mm was noted (Figure C15.2). The defect was noted to be contained with a well-defined transition zone and normal surrounding articular

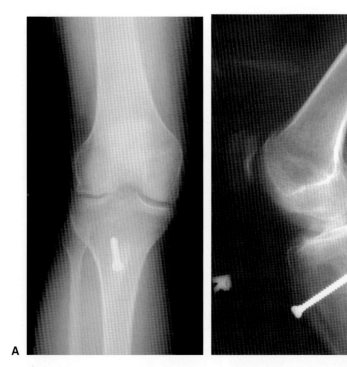

A   B

FIGURE C15.1. Preoperative anteroposterior (AP) **(A)** and lateral **(B)** radiographs of the right knee demonstrate fixation hardware from prior osteotomy procedure as well as flattening and irregularity of the lateral femoral condyle.

cartilage. An articular cartilage biopsy for future autologous chondrocyte implantation (ACI) was harvested from the intercondylar notch, in the same region as a notchplasty performed during anterior cruciate ligament (ACL) reconstruction is typically performed. Approximately 2 months later, the patient underwent ACI to the lateral femoral condyle lesion, which was noted to be 32 mm by 18 mm in dimension following debridement (Figure C15.3). Postoperatively, she was made heel-touch weight bearing for approximately 8 weeks and continued to use a continuous passive motion (CPM) machine for 6 to 8 h/day

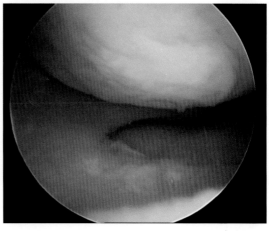

FIGURE C15.2. Arthroscopic photograph of the lateral femoral condyle of the right knee demonstrates large chondral defect filled with fibrocartilaginous tissue.

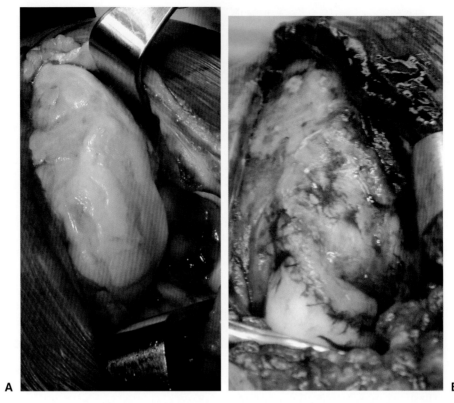

A   B

FIGURE C15.3. **(A)** Intraoperative photograph demonstrates large lateral femoral condyle lesion with full-thickness cartilage loss noted, with the central area filled with fibrocartilaginous tissue. **(B)** Lateral femoral condyle lesion with periosteal patch sewn in place, sealed by fibrin glue.

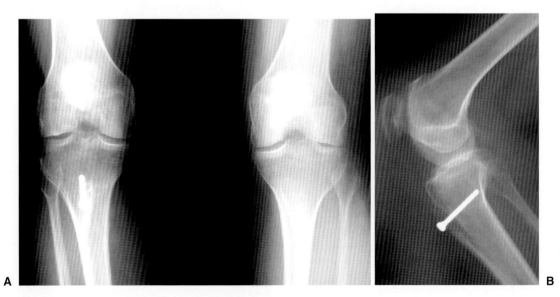

A   B

FIGURE C15.4. Twelve-month postoperative 45-degree posteroanterior flexion weight-bearing radiograph **(A)** and lateral radiograph **(B)** demonstrate slight improvement in the contour of the left lateral femoral condyle. No change in joint space is observed compared to preoperative radiographs.

for that same period of time. At 8 weeks, she was advanced to weight bearing and range of motion as tolerated. She advanced through the traditional rehabilitation protocol for ACI of the femoral condyle. She was asked to refrain from any impact or ballistic activities for 12 to 18 months.

FOLLOW-UP

The patient is now 18 months status post ACI. She states that she is totally painfree; however, she is still unable to fully perform high-impact activities due to muscular deconditioning. Her knee physical examination is entirely within normal limits. Radiographs obtained at 12 months demonstrate slight improvement in the contour of the lateral femoral condyle.

DECISION-MAKING FACTORS

1. Persistent symptoms despite several failed surgical attempts at patellar stabilization and loose body removal.
2. Young, high-demand patient with a large superficial chondral lesion amenable to chondrocyte transplantation or fresh osteochondral allograft. Lesion size precludes optimal result with microfracture or osteochondral autograft transplantation.
3. Patient preference for her own tissue and surgeon preference for ACI given the relatively young age of this patient and the desire to avoid the creation of a subchondral defect otherwise required for fresh osteochondral allograft transplantation.
4. Ability and willingness to be compliant with the postoperative course.

PATHOLOGY
Contained focal chondral defect of the medial femoral condyle

TREATMENT
Autologous chondrocyte implantation of the medial femoral condyle

SUBMITTED BY
Brian J. Cole, MD, MBA, Rush Cartilage Restoration Center, Rush University Medical Center, Chicago, Illinois, USA

CHIEF COMPLAINT AND HISTORY OF PRESENT ILLNESS

The patient is a 35-year-old woman who sustained a traumatic injury to her right knee while playing intramural softball 6 months before presenting for treatment. She complained of persistent medial joint line pain and activity-related swelling and effusions. She denied any giving-way or mechanical symptoms. Physical therapy failed to relieve her symptoms.

PHYSICAL EXAMINATION

Height, 5ft, 3in.; weight, 120lb. The patient ambulates with a nonantalgic gait. Her alignment is in slight symmetric valgus. She has full range of motion. A trace effusion is present with tenderness over the medial femoral condyle and medial joint line. Meniscal findings are present only on the medial side. Her ligament examination is normal.

RADIOGRAPHIC EVALUATION

Preoperative radiographs were within normal limits (Figure C16.1).

SURGICAL INTERVENTION

Due to her persistent symptoms, she was indicated for arthroscopy. At the time of arthroscopy, she was diagnosed as having a posterior horn medial meniscus tear involving approximately 20% of the medial meniscus as well as a grade IV focal chondral defect of the medial femoral condyle in the weight-bearing zone measuring approximately 25mm by 20mm (Figure C16.2). This lesion was simply debrided, and a concomitant articular cartilage biopsy was taken from the intercondylar notch. The patient did well initially with resolution of her medial joint line pain but complained of persistent weight-bearing discomfort. She continued to have activity-related effusions and

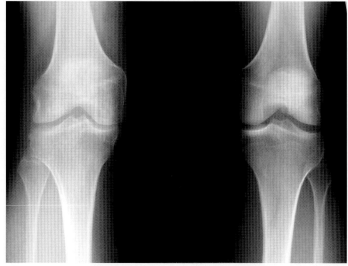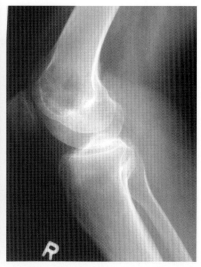

A   B

FIGURE C16.1. Posteroanterior 45-degree flexion weight-bearing **(A)** and lateral **(B)** radiographs obtained before index arthroscopy were essentially within normal limits save for some possible mild medial joint space narrowing.

complaints of discomfort with changes in barometric pressure. Because of her ongoing symptoms, the nature of her focal chondral defect, and the relatively small amount of previous medial meniscectomy, it was believed that the persistent symptoms were caused by the focal chondral defect. Thus, the patient underwent autologous chondrocyte implantation (ACI) (Figure C16.3).

Postoperatively, she was made nonweight bearing for approximately 4 weeks and subsequently advanced to full weight bearing. Additionally, during that time she used continuous passive motion for approximately 6 h/day. She advanced through the remainder of the rehabilitation protocol over the ensuing 12 months and was asked to refrain from impact activities for at least 12 months.

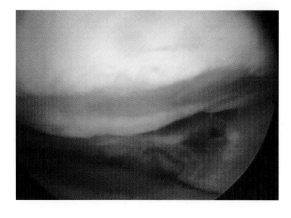

FIGURE C16.2. Arthroscopic photograph of a grade IV medial femoral condyle focal chondral defect obtained at the time of chondral debridement and partial medial meniscectomy.

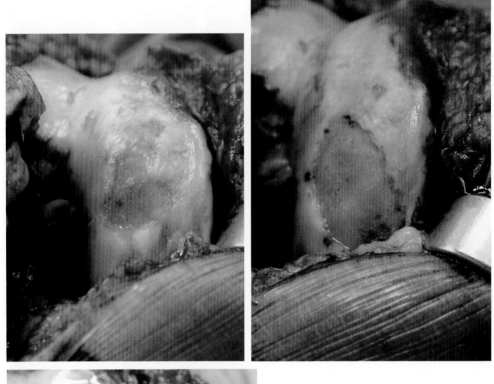

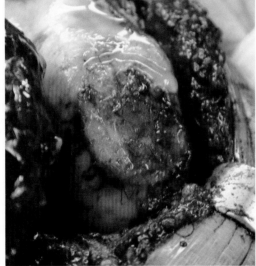

FIGURE C16.3. Clinical photographs at the time of autologous chondrocyte implantation demonstrate **(A)** the defect in the medial femoral condyle predebridement; **(B)** the defect postdebridement with vertical walls and no violation of the subchondral bone or calcified layer; and **(C)** the defect prepared with the periosteal patch sewn into place and fibrin glue applied.

FOLLOW-UP

She followed a fairly typical postoperative course but developed mechanical-type symptoms around the eighth postoperative month following autologous chondrocyte implanta-tion. Further efforts at rehabilitation failed, and the patient was indicated for a repeat arthroscopy 1 year postoperatively under the pretext that she may have periosteal patch detachment or hypertrophy. At the time of arthroscopy, the defect was well filled with soft,

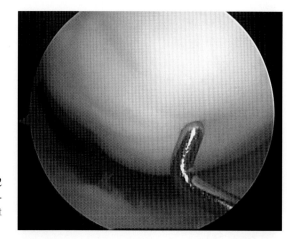

FIGURE C16.4. Second-look arthroscopy at 12 months demonstrates the defect filled and well integrated with hyaline-like tissue that is somewhat softer than the surrounding adjacent cartilage.

hyaline-like-appearing tissue with an unstable flap along the medial edge of the repair site (Figure C16.4). Indentation testing was performed that demonstrated that the implant was slightly softer than the normal native surrounding articular cartilage but still had a high degree of inherent stiffness (Figure C16.5). The region of periosteal delamination was debrided, and a 2-mm core biopsy was obtained for histologic evaluation (Figure C16.6). The

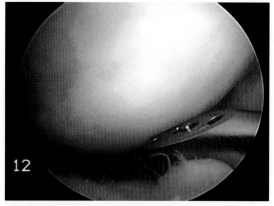

A

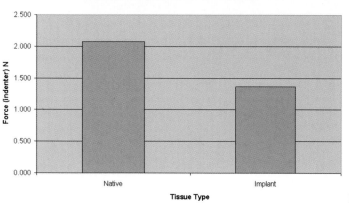

FIGURE C16.5. (A) Indentation testing is performed with evidence of a small area of periosteal detachment on the medial aspect of the defect. (B) Bar graph demonstrates the relative differences of the native articular cartilage compared to the hyaline-like tissue.

Native Articular Cartilage Stiffness vs ACI Implant at 1 Year

B

FIGURE C16.6. Safranin-O, fast green staining technique demonstrates variable degrees of proteoglycan staining within the deeper zones of the graft and integration of the hyaline-like tissue with the underlying subchondral bone. Magnification 4x original. (Courtesy of Dr. James M. Williams, PhD, Rush University.)

histologic evaluation demonstrated a well-integrated graft at the junction of the subchondral bone and variable amounts of proteoglycan production visibly decreasing from the subchondral bone junction toward the graft surface. Following this debridement, the patient went on to do well with no complaints of residual mechanical symptoms, minimal activity-related effusions, and has returned to intramural sports.

DECISION-MAKING FACTORS

1. Recurrent symptoms despite previous partial medial meniscectomy in a setting where the focal chondral defect was believed to initially represent an incidental finding requiring only simple debridement.
2. Persistent symptoms of pain and swelling in the exact location of the defect.
3. Normal alignment and ligament status with a defect measuring approximately $5\,cm^2$. As opposed to fresh osteochondral allograft transplantation, ACI performed in this relatively young patient will not compromise any future treatment options should they become necessary, that is, no violation of subchondral bone with ACI.

PATHOLOGY
Contained focal chondral defect of the medial femoral condyle

TREATMENT
Autologous chondrocyte implantation of the medial femoral condyle

SUBMITTED BY
Brian J. Cole, MD, MBA, Rush Cartilage Restoration Center, Rush University Medical Center, Chicago, Illinois, USA

CHIEF COMPLAINT AND HISTORY OF PRESENT ILLNESS

The patient is a 38-year-old man with a complaints of left knee medial-sided pain. Approximately 1 year before his initial presentation, he sustained a direct traumatic blow to the inner side of his left knee. He developed persistent weight-bearing pain and swelling. He underwent arthroscopy and was diagnosed with a grade IV medial femoral condyle focal chondral defect that was initially treated with abrasion arthroplasty at an outside institution (Figure C17.1). Postoperatively, the patient remained symptomatic with recurrent activity-related pain and effusions. He was unable to work as a waiter because of his persistent symptoms.

PHYSICAL EXAMINATION

Height, 5ft, 10in.; weight, 170lb. The patient ambulates with a significant antalgic gait. His alignment is in slight symmetric varus. He has full range of motion. He has significant tenderness over his medial femoral condyle and medial joint line. Meniscal compression signs are absent. He has mild medial tibiofemoral crepitus with passive range of motion. His ligament examination is normal.

RADIOGRAPHIC EVALUATION

Plain radiographs were within normal limits.

SURGICAL INTERVENTION

At the time of arthroscopy 1 year following his abrasion arthroplasty, he demonstrated soft fibrocartilage fill of a 25mm by 25mm medial femoral condyle defect with a firm base and palpable subchondral bone (Figure C17.2). At that time, it was elected to perform an articular cartilage biopsy from the intercondylar notch. Approximately 8 weeks later, the patient underwent autologous chondrocyte implantation (Figure C17.3). Postoperatively, he was made nonweight bearing for approximately 6 weeks and subsequently advanced to full weight bearing. Additionally, during that time he used continuous passive motion for approximately 6h/day. He advanced through the remainder of the rehabilitation protocol over the ensuing 12 months and had some difficulty regaining full flexion. He was asked to refrain from impact activities for at least 12 months.

FOLLOW-UP

The patient did well, and at 2 years follow-up he underwent repeat arthroscopy for a painful plica that was excised. At that time he had full

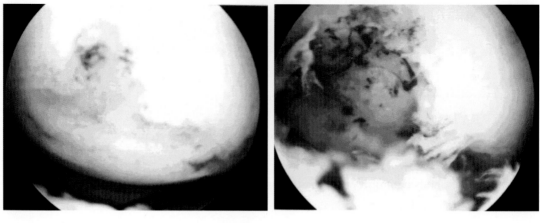

FIGURE C17.1. **(A)** Arthroscopic picture of the index defect of the medial femoral condyle. **(B)** Abrasion arthroplasty performed at the time of index surgery.

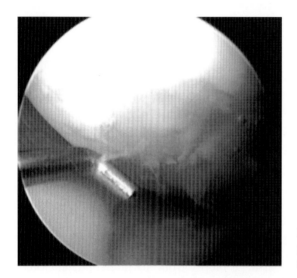

FIGURE C17.2. One-year postoperative arthroscopic picture demonstrates fibrocartilaginous fill that is soft with a firm, subchondral bed.

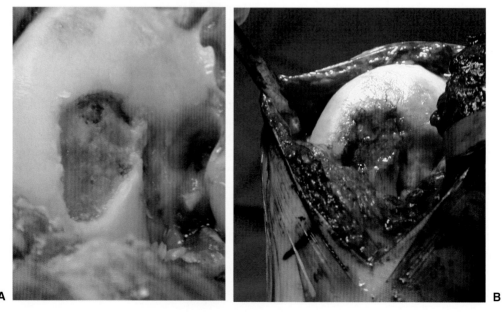

FIGURE C17.3. **(A)** Prepared defect of the medial femoral condyle measuring approximately 25 mm by 25 mm. **(B)** Periosteal patch sewn into place following fibrin glue placement.

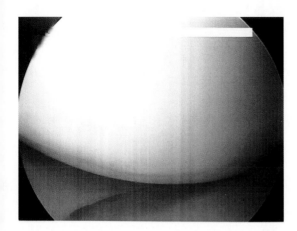

FIGURE C17.4. Second-look arthroscopy at 2 years demonstrates excellent fill with a smooth transition zone between the defect and normal surrounding articular cartilage.

range of motion with minimal tenderness over the defect, but complained of a palpable and painful catching sensation due to the plica. At the time of arthroscopic debridement, he was diagnosed as having excellent fill of the defect with hyaline-like cartilage that was palpably firm and had an excellent transition zone between it and the normal surrounding cartilage (Figure C17.4). The patient has returned to the workplace and complains of some difficulty with kneeling and squatting, with his most recent follow-up being 4 years following his index operation.

DECISION-MAKING FACTORS

1. Relatively young and active individual with a failure of a primary treatment attempt aimed at forming repair tissue within the defect.
2. Persistent symptoms of pain and swelling in the exact location of the defect.
3. A relatively contained lesion of appropriate size for autologous chondrocyte implantation offered as a second-line treatment option.
4. As opposed to fresh osteochondral allograft transplantation, ACI performed in this relatively young patient will not compromise any future treatment options should they become necessary, i.e., no violation of subchondral bone with ACI.

PATHOLOGY
Osteochondritis dissecans of the medial femoral condyle

TREATMENT
Autologous chondrocyte implantation of the medial femoral condyle

SUBMITTED BY
Brian J. Cole, MD, MBA, Rush Cartilage Restoration Center, Rush University Medical Center, Chicago, Illinois, USA

CHIEF COMPLAINT AND HISTORY OF PRESENT ILLNESS

This patient is a previously active 26-year-old man with a history of left knee problems dating back to approximately 14 months before his initial evaluation for cartilage restoration. His past history includes episodes of periodic swelling and locking, which led to an arthroscopic removal of a loose body emanating from a lesion of osteochondritis dissecans of the medial femoral condyle, performed approximately 12 months before this evaluation. The patient did well initially, but developed recurrent pain and swelling with weight-bearing activities and an inability to perform any impact or pivoting sports.

PHYSICAL EXAMINATION

Height, 6ft, 3in.; weight, 180lb. The patient walks with a nonantalgic gait. His standing alignment is in neutral. His left knee has a minimal effusion. His range of motion is 0 to 130 degrees. His medial femoral condyle is tender to palpation, and meniscal findings are absent. His ligament examination is within normal limits.

RADIOGRAPHIC EVALUATION

Initial radiographs demonstrate a lesion of osteochondritis dissecans in the typical zone of the medial femoral condyle of the left knee (Figure C18.1). Similarly, a magnetic resonance image (MRI) demonstrated loss of convexity of the medial femoral condyle in the region of the intercondylar notch with no evidence of a remaining fragment (Figure C18.2).

SURGICAL INTERVENTION

Because of his recurrent symptoms, the patient was indicated for arthroscopy and biopsy for autologous chondrocyte implantation (Figure C18.3). Approximately 5 weeks later, the patient underwent autologous chondrocyte implantation (ACI) (Figure C18.4). At the time of implantation, the lesion measured approximately 25mm in length, 22mm in width, and 6mm in depth. Postoperatively, the patient was made nonweight bearing for approximately 4 weeks and utilized continuous passive motion for 6 weeks at 6 to 8h/day. He advanced through the traditional rehabilitation protocol for ACI of the femoral condyle and was asked to refrain from any impact or ballistic activities for at least 12 months.

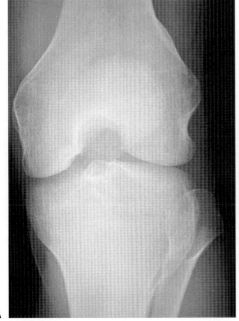 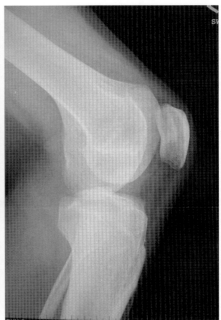

A   **B**

FIGURE C18.1. Preoperative posteroanterior 45-degree flexion weight-bearing **(A)** and lateral **(B)** radiographs demonstrate a lesion of osteochondritis dissecans in the typical zone of the medial femoral condyle of the left knee.

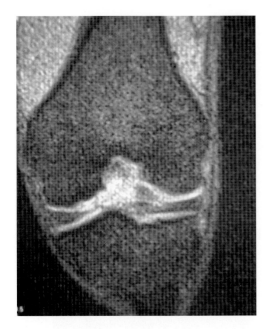 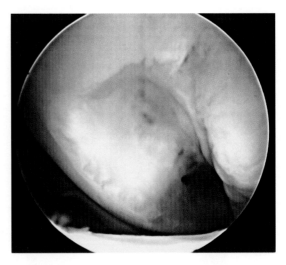

FIGURE C18.3. Arthroscopic photograph of the medial femoral condyle defect, taken at the time of biopsy.

FIGURE C18.2. MRI demonstrates loss of convexity of the medial femoral condyle in the region of the intercondylar notch with no evidence of remaining fragment.

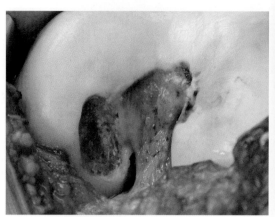
A

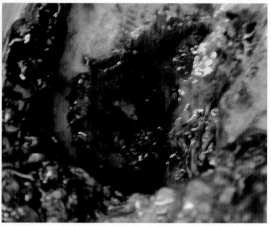
B

FIGURE C18.4. **(A)** Medial femoral condyle defect after preparation. The lesion measured approximately 25 mm in length, 22 mm in width, and 6 mm in depth. **(B)** After periosteal patch fixation.

FOLLOW-UP

At his 2-year follow-up visit he complained of no residual symptoms. He was participating in several high-level activities including running marathons and performing triathlons. Radiographs at that time demonstrated restoration of the medial femoral condyle in the previous region of osteochondritis dissecans with no evidence of sclerotic change, lucency, or joint space narrowing (Figure C18.5).

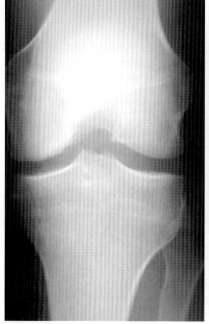
A

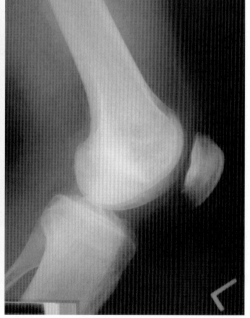
B

FIGURE 18.5. Two-year postoperative anteroposterior **(A)** and lateral **(B)** radiographs demonstrate restoration of the medial femoral condyle in the previous region of osteochondritis dissecans with no evidence of sclerotic change, lucency, or joint space narrowing.

DECISION-MAKING FACTORS

1. A failure of first-line treatment with persistent symptoms of activity-related weight-bearing pain in the region of the defect.
2. Young high-demand patient with symptomatic, relatively contained, shallow osteochondritis dissecans lesion considered relatively large for osteochondral autograft transplantation.
3. Patient preference for his own tissue and surgeon preference for ACI as a primary attempt at cartilage restoration to avoid creation of a deeper subchondral defect otherwise required for fresh osteochondral allograft transplantation.
4. Ability and willingness to be compliant with the postoperative course.

PATHOLOGY

Osteochondritis dissecans of the lateral femoral condyle

TREATMENT

Autologous chondrocyte implantation of the lateral femoral condyle

SUBMITTED BY

Brian J. Cole, MD, MBA, Rush Cartilage Restoration Center, Rush University Medical Center, Chicago, Illinois, USA

CHIEF COMPLAINT AND HISTORY OF PRESENT ILLNESS

The patient is a very active 19-year-old man who reports an injury to his right knee approximately 6 months prior while jumping from a fence. He subsequently developed the onset of sudden pain and swelling of his knee. He does recall occasional clicking before that time, but it became significantly worse after this recent traumatic event. Since the time of the injury, the patient has had weight-bearing discomfort with pain along the lateral aspect of his knee. He is unable to perform high-level activities because of the pain and activity-related swelling. Additionally, he reports a catching sensation. As a result of his present symptoms, he is unable to compete in intramural college athletics as he was able to do before this injury.

PHYSICAL EXAMINATION

Height, 5 ft, 8 in.; weight, 170 lb. The patient walks with a nonantalgic gait. His standing alignment is in symmetric physiologic varus. The right knee has a moderate effusion with positive lateral joint line tenderness, no medial joint line tenderness, and no varus or valgus instability upon stress testing. His lateral femoral condyle is painful to direct palpation. His ligament examination is within normal limits. He has full range of motion and has no meniscal findings.

RADIOGRAPHIC EVALUATION

Plain radiographs of the right knee including 45-degree flexion weight-bearing posteroanterior and nonweight-bearing lateral views reveal flattening of the lateral femoral condyle consistent with chronic osteochondritis dissecans. There appears to be minimal subchondral bone loss. Magnetic resonance imaging (MRI) is also consistent with the diagnosis of osteochondritis dissecans with minimal bony involvement (Figure C19.1).

SURGICAL INTERVENTION

Based on the patient's history, age, symptoms, physical examination, and radiographic studies, he was indicated for diagnostic arthroscopy, debridement of the lateral femoral condyle lesion, and possibly microfracture depending on the size and depth of the lesion. At arthroscopy, a grade IV 28 mm by 30 mm lesion of the lateral femoral condyle was noted. The lesion extended down to but not appreciably through the subchondral bone, and no loose bodies were identified (Figure C19.2). Because of the defect size, patient activity level, and

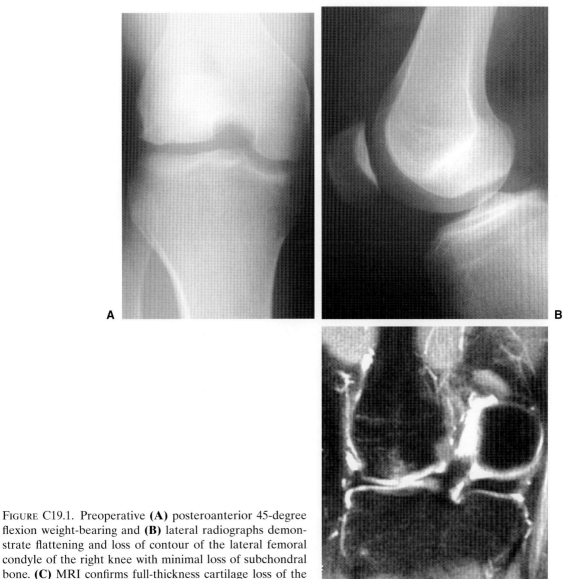

FIGURE C19.1. Preoperative **(A)** posteroanterior 45-degree flexion weight-bearing and **(B)** lateral radiographs demonstrate flattening and loss of contour of the lateral femoral condyle of the right knee with minimal loss of subchondral bone. **(C)** MRI confirms full-thickness cartilage loss of the lateral femoral condyle with minimal bony involvement.

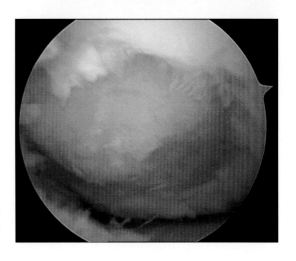

FIGURE C19.2. Arthroscopic photograph demonstrates grade IV lateral femoral condyle lesion measuring 28 mm by 30 mm, extending down to but not appreciably through the subchondral bone.

symptoms, it was elected to proceed with biopsy of the articular cartilage for eventual autologous chondrocyte implantation (ACI) and not to perform microfracture of the lesion.

The lesion was debrided, and a biopsy of 200 to 300 mg articular cartilage from the intercondylar notch was harvested. Approximately 2 months later, the patient returned and underwent ACI through a lateral-based arthrotomy (Figure C19.3). Postoperatively, the patient was made heel-touch weight bearing for 6 weeks and utilized continuous passive motion (CPM) for 6 to 8 h/day during that time. His range of motion was limited from full extension to 90

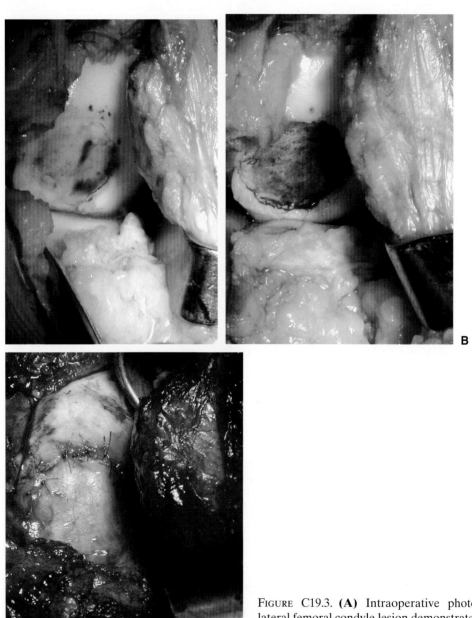

FIGURE C19.3. (A) Intraoperative photograph of the lateral femoral condyle lesion demonstrates full-thickness cartilage loss. (B) Lateral femoral condyle lesion after debridement. (C) Lateral femoral condyle lesion after the periosteal patch is sewn into place.

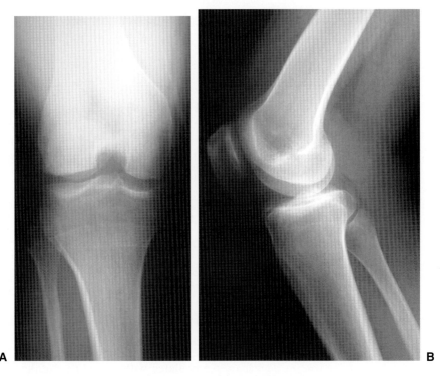

FIGURE C19.4. Postoperative anteroposterior **(A)** and lateral **(B)** radiographs at 1-year follow-up demonstrate good fill and contour of the lateral femoral condyle with no evidence of collapse.

degrees of flexion. At 6 weeks, weight bearing and range of motion were advanced as tolerated. He advanced through the traditional rehabilitation protocol for ACI of the femoral condyle and was asked to refrain from any impact or ballistic activities for at least 12 months.

FOLLOW-UP

The patient is now 24 months after ACI of the lateral femoral condyle of his right knee. He has no pain and has full range of motion. He runs, bikes, and skis on a regular basis. He is actively involved with intramural sports while attending college. His radiographs show early fill and restoration of contour of the lateral femoral condyle (Figure C19.4).

DECISION-MAKING FACTORS

1. Young, high-demand male with shallow osteochondritis dissecans lesion anticipated to be relatively unresponsive to microfracture and considered relatively large for osteochondral autograft transplantation.
2. Persistent symptoms of pain and swelling in the exact location of the defect.
3. Patient preference for his own tissue and surgeon preference for ACI as a primary cartilage restoration procedure given the relatively young age of this patient and the desire to avoid creating a subchondral defect otherwise required for fresh osteochondral allograft transplantation.
4. Ability and willingness to be compliant with the postoperative course.

PATHOLOGY
Uncontained focal chondral defect of the lateral trochlea

TREATMENT
Autologous chondrocyte implantation of the trochlea with distal realignment

SUBMITTED BY
Brian J. Cole, MD, MBA, Rush Cartilage Restoration Center, Rush University Medical Center, Chicago, Illinois, USA

CHIEF COMPLAINT AND HISTORY OF PRESENT ILLNESS

This patient is a 16-year-old girl with complaints of left knee pain and swelling of several years duration. She stated that her knee problems date back to when she was in the fourth grade at the age of 9 years. She sustained an injury that precipitated her symptoms, which have gradually worsened over the years. Two years previously, she underwent microfracture of an isolated chondral lesion of the trochlea due to her relentless symptoms of anterolateral knee pain and activity-related swelling. Initially, her symptoms were reduced. However, because of worsening complaints of swelling and pain over the ensuing 2 years, she presented for additional treatment. She indicates that although she thoroughly enjoys participating in sports, she has not been able to do so for the past few years as a result of severe knee pain. Furthermore, walking more than just a few blocks causes her knee pain and swelling, requiring her to rest and elevate her left leg. She is unable to perform stair climbing other than with a non-reciprocal gait due to severe anterolateral knee pain. Several months of aggressive patellofemoral rehabilitation failed to alleviate her symptoms.

PHYSICAL EXAMINATION

Height, 5ft, 5in.; weight, 122lb. The patient ambulates with a slightly antalgic gait on the left. Her standing alignment appears to be neutral and symmetric. A moderate effusion is present in the left knee. Her range of motion is from 0 to 135 degrees. She has 1cm of quadriceps atrophy when measured 10cm proximal to the patella. She has a full symmetric range of motion and mild patellar apprehension. She has mild lateral joint line tenderness, no medial joint line tenderness, and her meniscal findings are grossly absent. Additionally, she has 3+ crepitus of the patellofemoral joint with active extension. Her ligament examination is within normal limits.

RADIOGRAPHIC EVALUATION

Extension weight-bearing radiographs reveal some lateral femoral condyle flattening of the left knee. Overall, her alignment is normal with no evidence of degenerative changes or joint space narrowing (Figure C20.1). Merchant views demonstrated the patella to be centered within the trochlea and no evidence of trochlear hypoplasia. Given her well-documented history and consistent symptoms, no magnetic resonance imaging (MRI) was obtained.

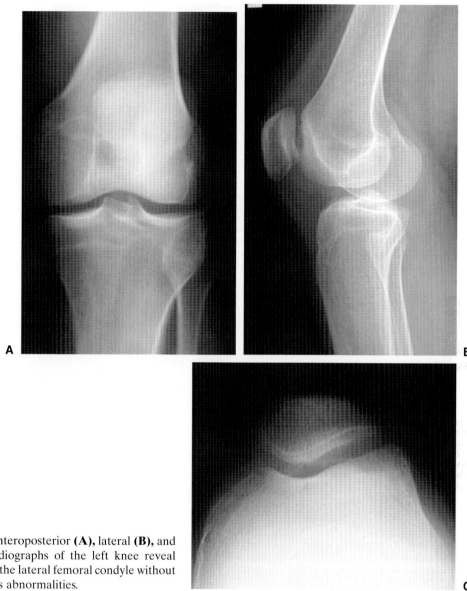

A

B

FIGURE C20.1. Anteroposterior **(A)**, lateral **(B)**, and merchant **(C)** radiographs of the left knee reveal mild flattening of the lateral femoral condyle without any other obvious abnormalities.

C

SURGICAL INTERVENTION

The patient underwent a left knee arthroscopy in which articular cartilage debridement was performed as well as a biopsy for autologous chondrocyte implantation (ACI). At the time of arthroscopy, a trochlear defect of approximately 30 mm by 35 mm was noted to be completely filled with soft fibrocartilage (Figure C20.2). The defect was laterally based with direct contact with the patella during the initial

phases of knee flexion. Approximately 2 months later, the patient underwent ACI of her chondral lesion in addition to a distal tibial tubercle anteromedialization procedure. Due to the uncontained nature of this laterally sided trochlear lesion, two mini suture-anchors were utilized to sew the periosteal patch to the periphery (Figures C20.3, C20.4). Additionally, juxtaarticular synovial tissue was utilized to help seal the periosteal patch. Postoperatively, she was made heel-touch weight bearing for

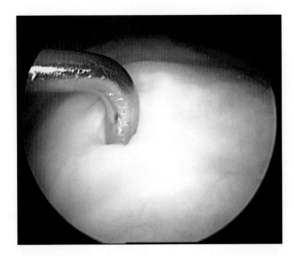

FIGURE C20.2. Arthroscopic probing of the trochlear lesion demonstrates a laterally based lesion with soft fibrocartilaginous repair tissue.

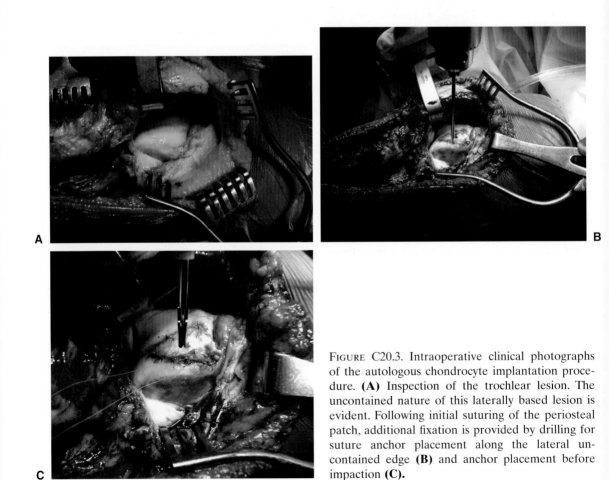

FIGURE C20.3. Intraoperative clinical photographs of the autologous chondrocyte implantation procedure. **(A)** Inspection of the trochlear lesion. The uncontained nature of this laterally based lesion is evident. Following initial suturing of the periosteal patch, additional fixation is provided by drilling for suture anchor placement along the lateral un-contained edge **(B)** and anchor placement before impaction **(C).**

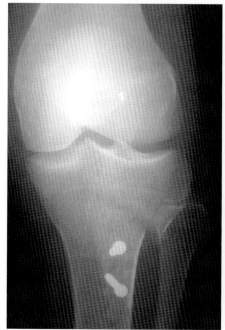
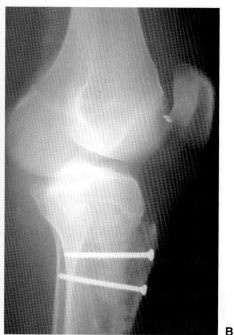

FIGURE C20.4. Postoperative anteroposterior **(A)** and lateral **(B)** radiographs of the left knee demonstrate the distal realignment procedure with hard-ware fixation in place. The two suture anchors utilized to secure the periosteal patch are also evident on these radiographic views.

approximately 6 weeks until radiographic healing of the distal realignment was demonstrated. She utilized continuous passive motion for 6 weeks initially with partial flexion restrictions. At 8 weeks, she was advanced to weight bearing and range of motion as tolerated. She advanced through the traditional rehabilitation protocol for ACI of the trochlea. She was asked to refrain from any impact or ballistic activities for 18 months.

FOLLOW-UP

At her 6-month follow-up visit, she ambulated without an antalgic gait, and her knee pain and swelling had decreased substantially. At 12 months, she was walking for long distances without pain. Stair climbing was virtually painfree. She has not begun participating in gym class or sports activities as yet. However, she believes that once the protocol permits, she would be symptom free enough to allow higher-level activities.

DECISION-MAKING FACTORS

1. Previously failed microfracture technique and aggressive physical therapy program emphasizing proper patellofemoral mechanics.
2. Young, high-demand patient without viable cartilage restoration alternatives.
3. Persistent symptoms of pain and swelling in the exact location of the defect.
4. Ability and willingness to be compliant with postoperative rehabilitation.

PATHOLOGY
Failed prior fresh osteochondral allograft of the medial femoral condyle

TREATMENT
Revision fresh osteochondral allograft with medial opening-wedge high tibial osteotomy and iliac crest bone graft

SUBMITTED BY
Brian J. Cole, MD, MBA, Rush Cartilage Restoration Center, Rush University Medical Center, Chicago, Illinois, USA

CHIEF COMPLAINT AND HISTORY OF PRESENT ILLNESS

The patient is an 18-year-old male who has had symptoms of bilateral knee pain for 5 years before his initial evaluation. His symptom onset was sudden, occurring while playing football. Two years previously, because of ongoing symptoms of osteochondritis dissecans of both medial femoral condyles, he underwent bilateral osteochondral allograft transplantation using fresh osteochondral allografts. The right knee was treated with an opening-wedge osteotomy due to a slight varus deformity, and the left knee, because of what was believed to be a minimal varus deformity, was left untreated without an osteotomy. The patient did well with respect to the right knee and became completely asymptomatic. However, his left knee remained symptomatic, with complaints of medial knee pain on a daily basis with weight-bearing activity-related swelling, stiffness, and inability to participate in sports. He has minimal mechanical symptoms. He would like to participate in intramural and high school level sports but is unable to do so.

PHYSICAL EXAMINATION

Height, 5 ft, 10 in.; weight, 190 lb. His gait is slightly antalgic on the left. The alignment reveals a slight varus deformity on the left and normal alignment to slight valgus on the right. There is a moderate effusion in the left knee. His range of motion is 0 to 130 degrees. He is tender along the medial femoral condyle and slightly tender along the joint line. Meniscal findings, however, are grossly absent. He has 2 cm of quadriceps atrophy in the left knee when measured 10 cm proximal to the patella. His ligament examination is normal.

RADIOGRAPHIC EVALUATION

Posteroanterior flexion weight-bearing radiographs demonstrate collapse of the medial femoral condyle osteochondral allograft of the left knee. The osteochondral allograft and high tibial osteotomy previously performed on the right knee are both well healed (Figure C21.1).

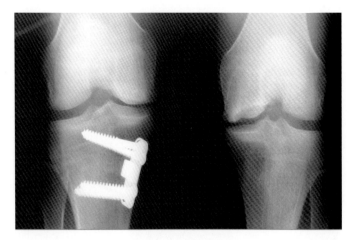

FIGURE C21.1. Flexion weight-bearing radiograph demonstrates collapse of the medial femoral condyle osteochondral allograft of the left knee and well-incorporated osteochondral allograft in the right knee with a well-healed osteotomy.

SURGICAL INTERVENTION

At the time of surgery on his left knee, there was a necrotic osteoarticular fragment and a defect measuring 30 mm by 30 mm by 8 mm in depth (Figure C21.2). The fragment was removed, and the patient underwent postoperative rehabilitation. Three months later, the patient underwent left knee osteochondral allograft reconstruction using a 30 mm by 30 mm fresh osteochondral allograft and a high tibial opening-wedge osteotomy with an 11-degree correction and iliac crest bone grafting (Figure C21.3). Postoperatively, he was made nonweight bearing for approximately 8 weeks. He utilized continuous passive motion and under-

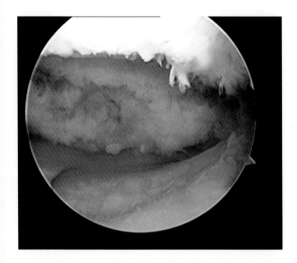

FIGURE C21.2. Arthroscopic view of the defect cavity within the medial femoral condyle following removal of the necrotic osteochondral allograft fragment.

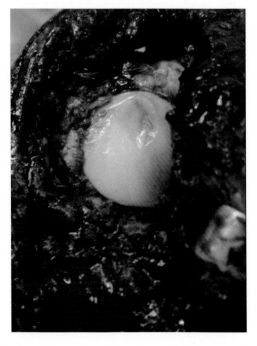

FIGURE C21.3. Intraoperative photograph of a 30 mm by 30 mm fresh osteochondral allograft placed within the medial femoral condyle.

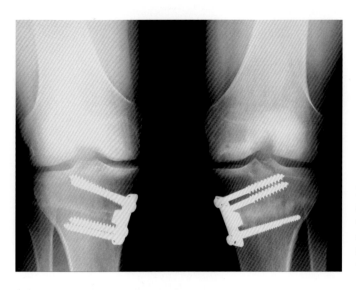

FIGURE 21.4. Eighteen-month radiograph demonstrates healing of the osteotomy and excellent incorporation of the medial femoral condyle osteochondral allograft with preservation of the medial joint space.

went progressive strengthening. At 8 weeks, he was advanced to weight bearing as tolerated. At 6 months, he was permitted to return to activities as tolerated.

FOLLOW-UP

At his 18-month follow-up visit, he demonstrated full range of motion, no swelling or pain, and had returned to all activities. Imaging studies reveal radiographic incorporation of his graft without collapse and a well-healed osteotomy (Figure C21.4). At the 3-year follow-up visit, he was completely asymptomatic.

DECISION-MAKING FACTORS

1. Young, active individual with symptoms related to lesion of osteochondritis dissecans.
2. Defect size greater than $3\,cm^2$ with subchondral bone loss beyond 6 to 8mm.
3. Failure of primary treatment with the possibility of biomechanical and biologic failure of the osteochondral allograft.
4. Contralateral knee with similar pathology successfully treated with combined fresh osteochondral allograft and opening-wedge high tibial osteotomy.

PATHOLOGY
Lateral meniscus deficiency

TREATMENT
Lateral meniscus allograft reconstruction

SUBMITTED BY
Brian J. Cole, MD, MBA, Rush Cartilage Restoration Center, Rush University Medical Center, Chicago, Illinois, USA

CHIEF COMPLAINT AND HISTORY OF PRESENT ILLNESS

This patient is an 18-year-old accomplished collegiate-level basketball player who presented following a lateral meniscectomy of her left knee performed 8 months previously, leaving her with persistent lateral joint line pain and activity-related swelling. These symptoms persisted despite having completed a rigorous postoperative physical therapy program. The symptoms occurred with routine activities and prevented her from playing basketball at a competitive level.

PHYSICAL EXAMINATION

Height, 5ft, 9in.; weight, 142lb. The patient ambulates with a nonantalgic gait. She stands in slight symmetric physiologic valgus. She has a moderate effusion. There is diffuse tenderness along the lateral joint line with pain created during placement of a valgus axial load. Her range of motion was symmetric to the contralateral side. There is approximately 2cm of quadriceps atrophy when compared to the contralateral side. She has no medial joint line tenderness and a normal ligamentous examination. There is no patellofemoral crepitus noted.

RADIOGRAPHIC EVALUATION

Plain radiographs show some flattening of the lateral femoral condyle of the left knee. There does not appear to be any bony deficit. There is no joint space narrowing, but definite irregularity is noted compared to the contralateral side.

SURGICAL INTERVENTION

Because of her persistent symptoms, she was indicated for a lateral meniscus allograft transplant. At surgery, it was noted that she had previously undergone a subtotal lateral meniscectomy and had minimal chondral change in that compartment (Figure C22.1A). Otherwise, the knee joint was within normal limits. A lateral meniscal transplant using a keyhole technique was performed (Figure C22.1B). Postoperative rehabilitation allowed weight bearing as tolerated up to 90 degrees of flexion, which remained restricted for the first 6 weeks. Return to unrestricted activities was permitted at 6 months.

FOLLOW-UP

The patient did well initially and, although she still had mild lateral joint line pain, it was much less than what she had experienced preopera-

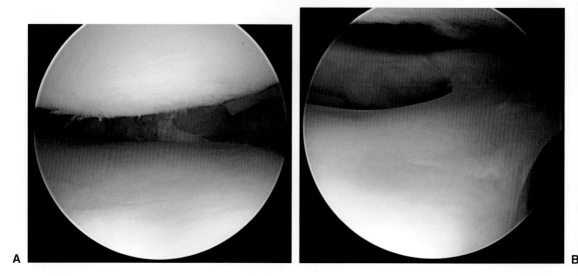

A   B

FIGURE C22.1. Arthroscopy of (A) the lateral compartment demonstrating prior subtotal meniscectomy and (B) the lateral meniscal transplant sutured into position.

tively. At 6 months postoperative, she was able to run for conditioning, but was not yet able to participate competitively. At 9 months postoperative, she developed occasional catching without any significant pain or swelling. She had full range of motion without evidence of lateral joint line pain. However, before being fully cleared for a return to basketball, a diagnostic arthroscopy was performed to assess for meniscal healing. At second-look arthroscopy, the repair was completely intact except for a small partial tear at the junction of the posterior horn and body, which was repaired using a formal inside-out technique (Figure C22.2). Subsequent to this procedure, the patient did quite well, and is now, 2.5 years after her lateral meniscus transplant, participating in all activities without limitations. Radiographs demonstrate no change in remaining joint space compared to her preoperative views (Figure C22.3).

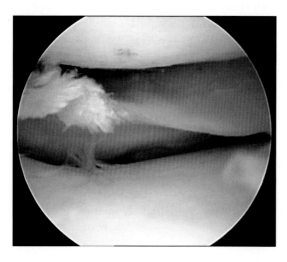

FIGURE C22.2. Arthroscopy at 9 months postoperatively shows an additional suture placed to repair a small area at the meniscal capsular junction believed to be contributing to the patient's persistent mechanical symptoms. Note the small area of degeneration at the posterior horn of the meniscus allograft.

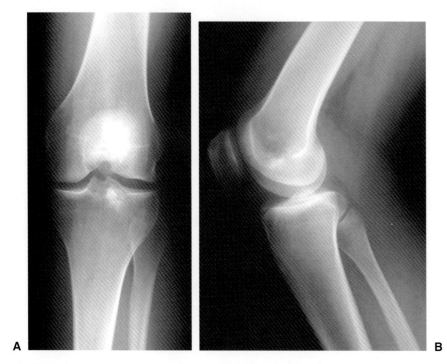

FIGURE C22.3. Two-year postoperative **(A)** anteroposterior and **(B)** lateral radiographs demonstrate maintenance of the lateral joint space with no evidence of collapse or degenerative changes.

DECISION-MAKING FACTORS

1. Young, active, high-demand patient with ipsilateral joint line symptoms following lateral meniscectomy.
2. Intact articular cartilage.
3. Demonstrated ability and understanding to adhere to rehabilitation protocol.
4. Unresponsiveness to meniscectomy and additional nonoperative treatment.

PATHOLOGY

Prior medial meniscectomy and focal chondral defect medial femoral condyle

TREATMENT

Medial meniscus allograft reconstruction with osteochondral autograft transplantation

SUBMITTED BY

Brian J. Cole, MD, MBA, Rush Cartilage Restoration Center, Rush University Medical Center, Chicago, Illinois, USA

CHIEF COMPLAINT AND HISTORY OF PRESENT ILLNESS

The patient is a 40-year-old woman who had a previous medial meniscectomy of the left knee, after which she did well for approximately 5 years. She presents with moderate to severe weight-bearing pain and medial joint line discomfort. She is unable to walk more than two blocks before having to stop due to increasing discomfort. She complains of pain at night when the inner side of her knees rest against each other. Initial treatment included physical therapy and a cortisone injection that provided no relief of her symptoms.

PHYSICAL EXAMINATION

Height, 5 ft, 6 in.; weight, 130 lb. The patient walks with a slightly antalgic gait. Her left knee is in neutral alignment compared to the right knee, which is in slight physiologic valgus. The left knee has a small effusion. She has full symmetric range of motion. Her medial femoral condyle and joint line are both tender to palpation. She has full range of motion, no patellofemoral crepitus, and a normal ligament examination.

RADIOGRAPHIC EVALUATION

Preoperative radiographs demonstrate mild medial joint space narrowing with no significant flattening of the medial femoral condyle (Figure C23.1).

SURGICAL INTERVENTION

At the time of cartilage restoration surgery (Figure C23.2), she was identified as having a previous subtotal medial meniscectomy and an associated grade IV focal chondral defect along the medial femoral condyle measuring approximately 10 mm by 10 mm. She underwent allograft medial meniscus transplantation using a double bone plug technique and osteochondral autograft transplantation using a single 10-mm-diameter plug (Figure C23.3). Postoperative rehabilitation included partial weight bearing for the first 4 weeks with immediate use of continuous passive motion for 6 h/day for the first 6

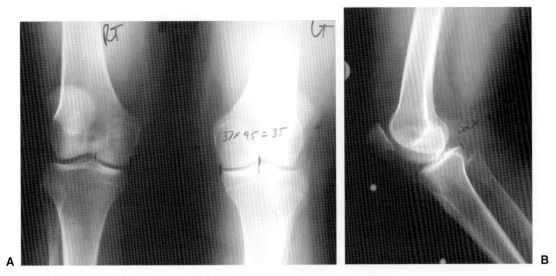

FIGURE C23.1. Extension weight-bearing anteroposterior **(A)** and lateral **(B)** radiographs demonstrate mild medial joint space narrowing without flattening of the femoral condyle or significant osteophyte formation.

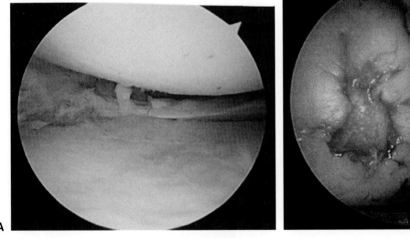
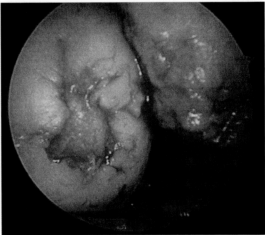

FIGURE C23.2. **(A)** Arthroscopic photograph obtained at the time of meniscus transplantation demonstrates prior subtotal medial meniscectomy with minimal changes in the articular surface of the tibia. **(B)** Arthroscopic photograph taken through the arthrotomy shows the 10 mm by 10 mm grade IV defect of the medial femoral condyle.

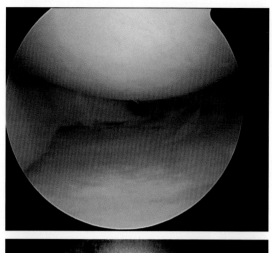

A

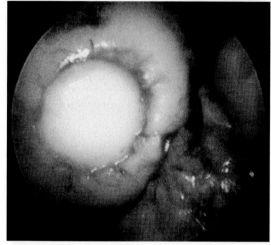

B

FIGURE C23.3. **(A)** Allograft medial meniscus transplant sutured in place. **(B)** The 10-mm-diameter osteochondral autograft is in place, effectively resurfacing the medial femoral condyle defect.

weeks. Return to unrestricted activities was permitted at 6 months.

FOLLOW-UP

At the 2-year follow-up visit, she demonstrates no progression of joint space narrowing and excellent integration of the osteochondral plug (Figure C23.4). She returned to all activities with no complaints of pain or swelling.

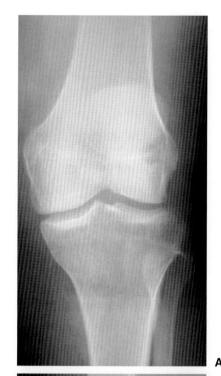

A

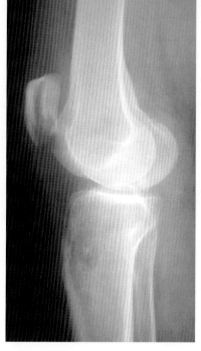

B

FIGURE C23.4. Two-year postoperative anteroposterior **(A)** and lateral **(B)** radiographs demonstrate preservation of joint space with no progression in degeneration and full integration of the osteochondral allograft plug with no cystic change or collapse.

DECISION-MAKING FACTORS

1. Active patient in her fifth decade with ipsilateral symptoms believed to be related to a prior subtotal meniscectomy and, possibly, to the associated defect of her medial femoral condyle.
2. Concomitant pathology requiring simultaneous treatment to eliminate any contraindication to either procedure being performed in isolation.
3. Absence of contraindications to meniscus transplantation including the lack of significant malalignment, the absence of bipolar disease, and a correctable grade IV lesion of the medial femoral condyle.
4. Relatively small defect (less than or equal to approximately $1\,cm^2$) with a single stage solution that will restore the surface with hyaline cartilage.

PATHOLOGY
Failed anterior cruciate ligament reconstruction with medial meniscus deficiency

TREATMENT
Revision anterior cruciate ligament reconstruction and medial meniscus allograft reconstruction

SUBMITTED BY
Brian J. Cole, MD, MBA, Rush Cartilage Restoration Center, Rush University Medical Center, Chicago, Illinois, USA

CHIEF COMPLAINT AND HISTORY OF PRESENT ILLNESS

This 16-year-old male patient is a high school soccer player who sustained a complete tear of his anterior cruciate ligament (ACL) during a soccer game approximately 18 months before presentation. He underwent ACL reconstruction using a bone–patella tendonbone autograft. His postoperative course was uncomplicated; he had complete relief of his pain and instability, and was able to return to playing competitive soccer. Approximately 11 months later, while playing soccer he felt a pop in his knee. He came to arthroscopic evaluation, at which time he was noted to have a large irreparable bucket-handle tear of his medial meniscus that required a subtotal meniscectomy. Although still intact, the ACL graft was probed and believed to be lax. At the time of presentation for cartilage restoration, he complained of persistent medial-sided knee pain, repeated giving-way, and activity-related effusions.

PHYSICAL EXAMINATION

Height, 5 ft, 10 in.; weight, 145 lb. The patient walks with a nonantalgic gait. He stands in neutral alignment. His range of motion is symmetric to the contralateral knee without any prone heel height difference. He has a trace effusion. He has significant tenderness along the medial joint line. The Lachman examination is grade II with firm endpoints, and he has a grade I to II pivot shift. His KT-2000 test reveals an 8-mm side-to-side difference on maximum manual testing. He has no posterior drop-back or sag, and he has no increased external rotation with manual testing. The remainder of his examination is unremarkable.

RADIOGRAPHIC EVALUATION

Plain radiographs including flexion weight-bearing and lateral views of the left knee reveal no evidence of joint space narrowing. The bone tunnels from prior ACL reconstruction are appropriately positioned, and a fixation screw is noted on the tibial side (Figure C24.1A,B). Magnetic resonance imaging (MRI) examination reveals almost complete absence of the medial meniscus, with no subchondral edema and intact articular cartilage (Figure C24.1C).

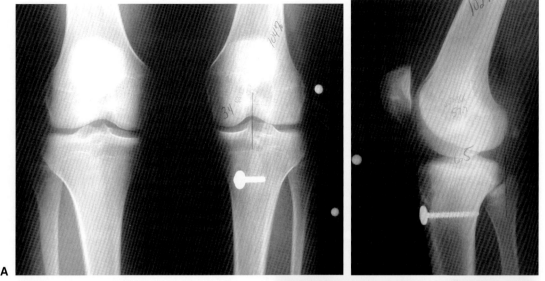

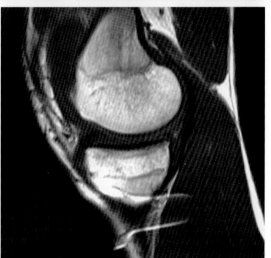

FIGURE C24.1. Sizing X-rays obtained to plan for meniscal allograft reconstruction. Weight-bearing anteroposterior **(A)** and lateral **(B)** radiographs of the left knee demonstrate preservation of the joint space as well as prior anterior cruciate ligament (ACL) fixation in good position. **(C)** MRI reveals almost complete absence of the medial meniscus.

SURGICAL INTERVENTION

The patient was indicated for simultaneously performed left knee medial meniscus allograft transplantation and revision ACL reconstruction with bone–patellar tendon–bone allograft. The principal indications for this simultaneous procedure included ipsilateral post-meniscectomy pain and recurrent ACL insufficiency. The primary indications for allograft meniscus transplantation included pain and instability, with consideration given to the role of the posterior horn of the medial meniscus as a secondary stabilizer to anterior translation. At the time of

surgery, the ACL was lax to probing and believed to be attenuated (Figure C24.2A). Inspection of the medial joint space revealed near absence of the entire medial meniscus with relatively intact articular cartilage (Figure C24.2B).

The medial meniscus allograft was prepared using a double-bone plug technique. A 10-mm-wide bone–patellar tendon–bone allograft was fashioned with two 10mm by 25mm bone blocks (Figure C24.2C). The posterior horn tunnel for the medial meniscus was drilled first, followed by the tibial and femoral tunnels, respectively, for the ACL. The medial meniscus was introduced and secured with vertical

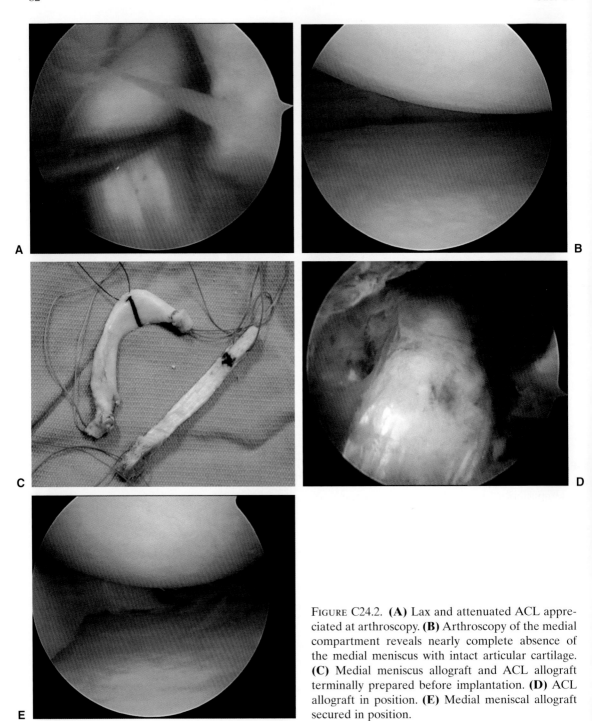

FIGURE C24.2. **(A)** Lax and attenuated ACL appreciated at arthroscopy. **(B)** Arthroscopy of the medial compartment reveals nearly complete absence of the medial meniscus with intact articular cartilage. **(C)** Medial meniscus allograft and ACL allograft terminally prepared before implantation. **(D)** ACL allograft in position. **(E)** Medial meniscal allograft secured in position.

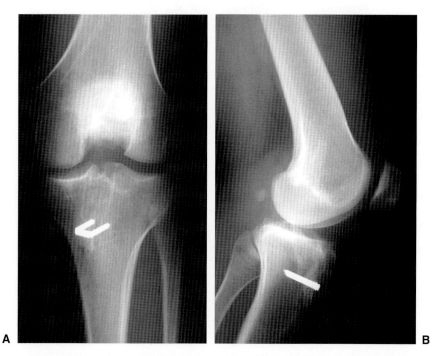

A   **B**

FIGURE C24.3. Posteroanterior 45-degree flexion weight-bearing (**A**) and lateral (**B**) radiograph obtained 14 months after allograft medial meniscus transplantation and revision ACL reconstruction.

mattress sutures and seating of the posterior bone plug into its recipient tunnel. The anterior horn was fixed into a blind tunnel at the anatomic insertion of the native meniscus insertion site. Finally, the ACL was passed and secured with a staple on the tibia and a ligament button on the femur due to slight graft mismatch and partial compromise of the posterior cortex of the femur (Figure C24.2D,E). Postoperative rehabilitation was guided primarily by the ACL protocol except for restriction of weight bearing beyond 90 degrees of knee flexion for the first 6 weeks. Return to unrestricted activities was permitted at 6 months.

FOLLOW-UP

At 18 months, the patient had full range of motion, denied any medial-sided knee pain, and had no complaints of instability. He had a grade I Lachman examination with a firm endpoint and a negligible pivot shift. Radiographs demonstrated excellent positioning of the ACL graft and proper seating of the meniscus transplant bone plugs. No evidence of joint space

narrowing was present (Figure C24.3). Repeat KT-2000 evaluation revealed a 2-mm side-to-side difference on maximum manual testing. The patient recently returned to participating in competitive soccer.

DECISION-MAKING FACTORS

1. Young, high-demand patient with ipsilateral symptoms related to a prior subtotal meniscectomy with a chief complaint of pain and instability.
2. Loss of the primary (ACL) and secondary (posterior horn of the medial meniscus) restraints to anterior translation of the left knee.
3. Intact articular cartilage.
4. A relative contraindication to performing an isolated medial meniscus transplant without ACL reconstruction. Similarly, revision ACL reconstruction without improving the secondary restraints for anterior tibial translation may place the newly reconstructed ACL at continued risk for premature failure.

PATHOLOGY
Advanced patellofemoral arthritis

TREATMENT
Patellofemoral arthroplasty

SUBMITTED BY
Tom Minas, MD, and Tim Bryant, RN, Cartilage Repair Center, Brigham and Women's Hospital, Chestnut Hill, Massachusetts, USA

CHIEF COMPLAINT AND HISTORY OF PRESENT ILLNESS

The patient is a 41-year-old man with a long-standing history of anterior right knee pain. As a teenager he sustained a patellar dislocation with an osteoarticular fracture. An open VMO quadriceps repair and removal of loose body was performed. Since then, five further arthroscopic debridements have been performed. Presently he complains of chronic right anterior knee pain. He uses antiinflammatories and ice for pain management only. He has pain that awakens him at night when he rolls over in bed. He is able to walk better on level surfaces than on inclines or up and down stairs. Additionally, he must use a handrail one step at a time to ascend or descend the stairs. He has frequent activity-related effusions. He requests a definitive operation that will relieve him of his pain and allow him to rapidly return to work to support his family. His job does not require physical or labor-intensive activities.

PHYSICAL EXAMINATION

Height, 6 ft, 1 in.; weight, 210 lb. Clinical examination demonstrates a relatively fit 41-year-old man with clinically neutral alignment. He walks with an antalgic gait. He must use his hands to get out of a seated position; he is unable to crouch or squat. His range of motion is from 0 to 125 degrees of flexion. Other findings include severe patellofemoral crepitation, a large joint effusion, and a relatively normal quadriceps angle of 15 degrees. His ligament and meniscal examination is unremarkable.

RADIOGRAPHIC EVALUATION

Standing radiographs demonstrate a well-maintained tibiofemoral joint space. Radiographs demonstrate a narrowed patellofemoral joint space (Figure C25.1).

SURGICAL INTERVENTION

At arthrotomy, the tibiofemoral articulations were intact. The patellofemoral joint demonstrated severe erosive grade IV changes to the trochlea and the patella with a convex hypoplastic trochlea (Figure C25.2). A patellofemoral arthroplasty was performed (Figure C25.3). Postoperatively, the patient advanced readily to weight bearing and range of motion as tolerated.

FOLLOW-UP

Within 3 weeks of his patellofemoral prosthesis, the patient was pain free and returned to work. Two years after implantation, he remains satisfied with the result.

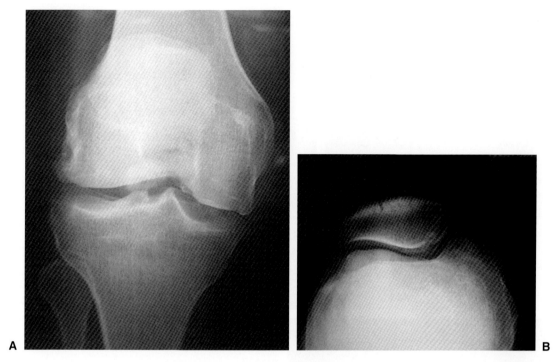

FIGURE C25.1. Preoperative plain standing anteroposterior **(A)** and skyline **(B)** radiographs demonstrate normal tibiofemoral joint space with central and lateral patellofemoral compartment joint space narrowing.

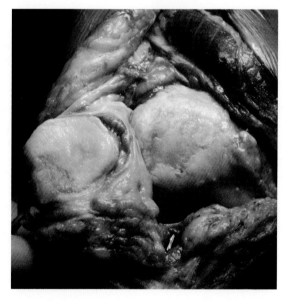

FIGURE C25.2. Appearance at the time of open arthrotomy. The trochlea is convex, hypoplastic, and has severe erosive changes. Similarly, the patella has a large area of exposed bone and has a dysplastic concave appearance.

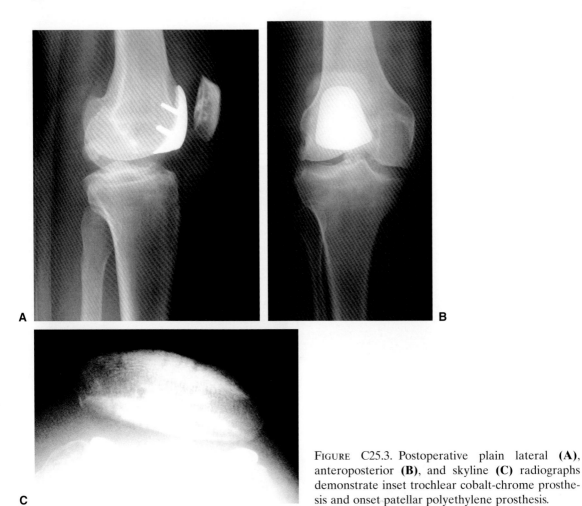

FIGURE C25.3. Postoperative plain lateral **(A)**, anteroposterior **(B)**, and skyline **(C)** radiographs demonstrate inset trochlear cobalt-chrome prosthesis and onset patellar polyethylene prosthesis.

DECISION-MAKING FACTORS

1. Advanced, highly symptomatic, isolated patellofemoral arthritis unresponsive to prior efforts at debridement and conservative management.
2. Disease extent poses a highly guarded prognosis for autologous chondrocyte implantation (ACI). Although osteochondral allograft remains a viable treatment option, it also carries a more guarded prognosis, and the patient is unwilling to undergo the prolonged rehabilitation required of this cartilage transplantation procedure.
3. A willingness to maintain relatively reduced activity levels to maximize the longevity of patellofemoral arthroplasty. The patient desires a predictable outcome and has low-demand requirements.
4. Informed consent that should the patellofemoral arthroplasty fail, revision to total knee arthroplasty is unlikely to be compromised.

PATHOLOGY
Multiple chondral defects

TREATMENT
Autologous chondrocyte implantation of the trochlea and medial and lateral femoral condyles

SUBMITTED BY
Jack Farr, MD, Cartilage Restoration Center of Indiana, OrthoIndy, Indianapolis, Indiana, USA

CHIEF COMPLAINT AND HISTORY OF PRESENT ILLNESS

This patient is a 43-year-old man with a 10-year history of lateral- greater than medial-sided knee pain as well as anterior knee pain. He complains of catching and effusions in his right knee. At the time of evaluation, he provided a history of having undergone arthroscopic treatment previously that provided minimal relief of his symptoms. The patient works as a full-time firefighter and complained of difficulty performing all his duties because of activity-related pain. His desire is to return to higher levels of activity that he previously enjoyed, including jogging and racquetball. At the time of initial presentation, he limited his activities to golf and biking and had gained 40 lb during the previous 2 years.

Review of the operative record indicates that 6 years previously he underwent chondroplasty and drilling of his femoral condyle. A repeat chondroplasty and drilling was performed 1 year before presentation. Despite these treatments, his symptoms recurred.

PHYSICAL EXAMINATION

Height, 5 ft, 9 in.; weight, 228 lb. The patient stands in slight varus alignment compared to neutral on the contralateral limb. He ambulates with a slightly antalgic gait on the right. He has a trace effusion. He has no gross atrophy. His range of motion is 0 to 130 degrees on the right compared to 0 to 135 degrees on the left. His ligament exam is unremarkable. He has marked tenderness on the lateral joint line and, to a lesser degree, at the medial joint line and patellofemoral joint. There are no mechanical signs, and patellar tracking is normal.

RADIOGRAPHIC EVALUATION

Weight-bearing anteroposterior and lateral radiographs show slight medial joint space narrowing and ossification changes in the lateral femoral condyle (due to prior drilling) (Figure C26.1). The Merchant view shows the patella to be centrally located. His long-leg alignment views show only 2 degrees of varus compared to the contralateral side. His magnetic resonance image (MRI) is consistent with a chronic osteochondritis dissecans of the lateral femoral condyle and chondrosis of the medial and patellofemoral compartments.

SURGICAL INTERVENTION

At the time of staging arthroscopy and biopsy for autologous chondrocyte implantation (ACI), grade IV chondrosis was noted at the trochlea (2.0 cm by 3.0 cm), medial (1.5 cm by 2.0 cm), and lateral (1.2 cm by 1.1 cm) femoral condyles (Figure C26.2). These lesions were contained. The opposing articular cartilage was intact. At the time of definitive treatment, ACI was performed for all three lesions (Figure C26.3). No realignment was performed.

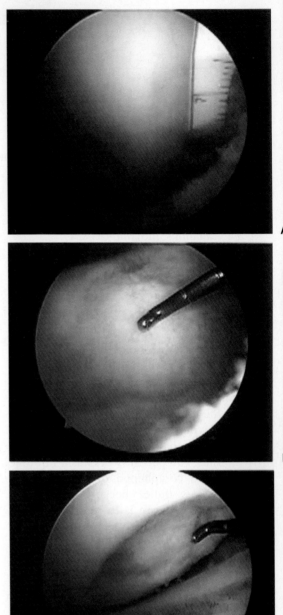

FIGURE C26.2. At index arthroscopy, lesions of the **(A)** medial femoral condyle, **(B)** trochlea, and **(C)** lateral femoral condyle are visualized.

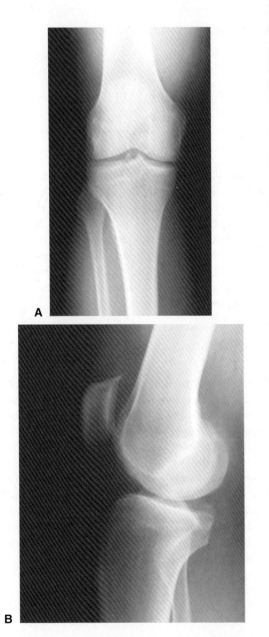

FIGURE C26.1. Anteroposterior **(A)** and lateral **(B)** radiographs demonstrate maintenance of joint spaces.

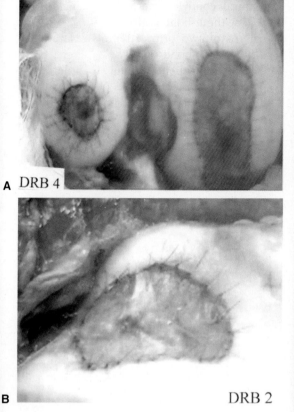

A DRB 4

B DRB 2

FIGURE C26.3. Autologous chondrocyte implantation (ACI) periosteal patches in place: **(A)** medial and lateral femoral condyles and **(B)** trochlea.

Postoperatively, the patient was made protected weight bearing with crutches for 6 weeks and utilized continuous passive motion for 3 weeks initially with restricted motion. The patient slowly advanced to full, unrestricted activities by 18 months.

FOLLOW-UP

The patient had returned to high-level activities including full-time firefighting. Second-look arthroscopy 3 years following the implantation revealed excellent fill and marginal integration of all defects (Figure C26.4).

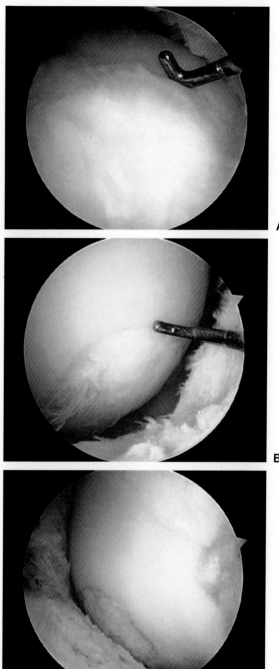

A

B

C

FIGURE C26.4. Second-look arthroscopy demonstrates excellent fill and marginal integration of **(A)** trochlea, **(B)** medial femoral condyle, and **(C)** lateral femoral condyle.

DECISION-MAKING FACTORS

1. Active patient with multiple focal chondral defects with limited alternatives to ACI, especially because of the concomitant symptomatic trochlear defect.
2. Despite a mild varus deformity, the presence of lateral compartment disease led to the decision to avoid osteotomy.
3. Shallow osteochondral lesion of the lateral femoral condyle amenable to single-stage ACI without bone grafting.
4. Failure of two prior attempts at standard drilling and chondroplasty.
5. Compliant patient willing to tolerate a prolonged rehabilitation period with a desire to return to high-level activities if possible.

PATHOLOGY
Traumatic patellar instability with focal chondral defect of the patella

TREATMENT
Autologous chondrocyte implantation of the patella with distal realignment (Note that the use of ACI for the patella is considered off-label usage, but was indicated and performed with explicit patient and family informed consent and under the guidance of an Institutional Review Board protocol allowing prospective study of this patient at the author's institution.)

SUBMITTED BY
Brian J. Cole, MD, MBA, Rush Cartilage Restoration Center, Rush University Medical Center, Chicago, Illinois, USA

CHIEF COMPLAINT AND HISTORY OF PRESENT ILLNESS

The patient is a 17-year-old female who initially presented with a 3-year history of left knee problems. She first injured her knee while playing basketball when she dislocated her patella. She complains of anterior left knee pain, giving-way, catching of the patellofemoral joint, and residual symptoms consistent with patellar instability. Her symptoms have been getting progressively worse. She rates her overall knee function as being poor and states that before her injury her knee was nearly normal. Previously, she had undergone an arthroscopy during which a small osteochondral lesion of the patella was noted. A 1.5-cm loose body was found and removed. The loose piece was derived from the patella, leaving a full-thickness cartilage lesion of the patella approximately 1.5 cm in diameter with minimal bone loss. At the time of loose body removal, a lateral release was performed. She underwent extensive physical therapy, emphasizing a patellofemoral rehabilitation program. Before this injury, she was a very active adolescent girl participating in multiple sports at her school. At the time of presentation, she was unable to participate in any sports because of her significant knee-related complaints.

PHYSICAL EXAMINATION

Height, 5 ft, 2 in.; weight, 105 lb. The patient ambulates with a nonantalgic gait. She stands in approximately 4 degrees of symmetric mechanical-axis valgus. She has a mild bilateral pronation deformity of both hindfeet. She has a moderate-sized joint effusion. She has significant patellar apprehension with two-quadrant laxity medially and three-quadrant laxity laterally. There is no excessive patellar tilt or subluxation when measured passively. She has a positive J sign and a Q angle of 10 degrees. She has crepitus with active flexion and extension with an audible and palpable catching sensation of the patella at approximately 45 degrees of flexion. The medial and lateral joint lines are not painful. Her ligament examination is within normal limits.

RADIOGRAPHIC EVALUATION

Plain radiographs revealed no significant sub-chondral sclerosis or joint space narrowing, but did reveal a definite central irregularity of the patella best seen on the lateral view. Merchant views demonstrated the patella to be centered within the trochlea. There was no evidence of trochlear hypoplasia. Magnetic resonance images demonstrate a central patellar chondral defect with slight edema in the subchondral bone in the region of the defect.

SURGICAL INTERVENTION

The patient underwent her second left knee arthroscopy during which a full-thickness chondral defect was noted in the central aspect of the patella measuring approximately 16 mm by 16 mm (Figure C27.1). At the same time, an articular cartilage biopsy was performed with the intention to perform autologous chondrocyte implantation (ACI) of the patella within 3 months of this intervention.

Approximately 10 weeks later, the patient underwent ACI through a lateral arthrotomy

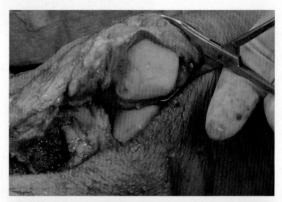

A

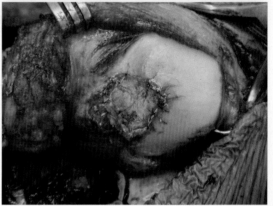

B

FIGURE C27.2. Intraoperative photographs at the time of autologous chondrocyte implantation procedure. Patellar lesion before (A) and after (B) the periosteal patch is sewn in place.

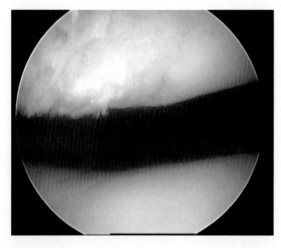

FIGURE C27.1. Arthroscopic photograph reveals full-thickness chondral defect of the patella measuring approximately 16 mm by 16 mm in diameter.

centered over the lateral retinaculum (Figure C27.2). A concomitant distal realignment procedure was also performed (Figure C27.3). The patellar defect was essentially central and circular, measuring 16 mm by 16 mm with minimal bony involvement. Postoperatively, she was made heel-touch weight bearing for approximately 6 weeks until radiographs demonstrated evidence of healing of the distal realignment. Although she was allowed to flex her knee daily to 90 degrees, continuous passive motion was restricted to 45 to 60 degrees of flexion during its use for the first 6 postoperative weeks. She advanced through the traditional rehabilitation protocol for ACI of the patella. She was asked

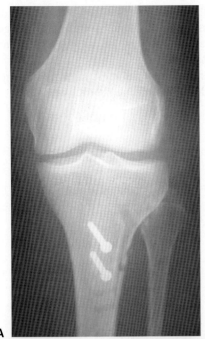

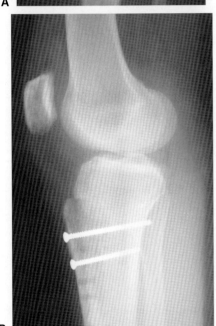

A

B

Figure C27.3. Postoperative anteroposterior (A) and lateral (B) radiographs reveal anteromedialization osteotomy of the tibial tubercle.

to refrain from any impact or ballistic activities for 18 months.

FOLLOW-UP

Four months following ACI of her patella, with the exception of open-chain kinetic exercise, she remained painfree. Additionally, there was no visible swelling. Her motion was symmetric bilaterally, ranging from 0 degrees of extension to 140 degrees of flexion. The catching sensation she experienced preoperatively was eliminated by 6 months. Because of some discomfort related to the screws placed to secure the distal realignment, she underwent second-look arthroscopy at 12 months (Figure C27.4) and hardware removal. At 2 years postoperatively, she continues to do well with respect to her anterior knee pain and is very satisfied with the results of her surgery. She regularly engages in high-level activities that include running and soccer.

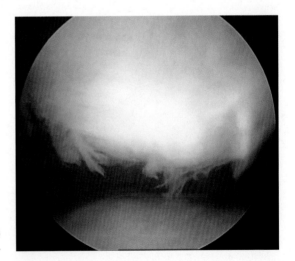

Figure C27.4. Second-look arthroscopy at 12 months performed during screw removal from the healed tibial tubercle osteotomy. Defect is filled with firm hyaline-like cartilage with some superficial fibrillation. Integration is good with no areas of exposed bone or delamination.

DECISION-MAKING FACTORS

1. Previously failed arthroscopic debridement and aggressive physical therapy program emphasizing proper patellofemoral mechanics.
2. Young, high-demand patient without viable cartilage restoration alternatives.
3. Full-thickness patellar chondral defect causing pain and swelling with mechanical symptoms in addition to patellar instability.
4. Ability and willingness to remain compliant with postoperative rehabilitation.

PATHOLOGY
Focal chondral defect patella

TREATMENT
Autologous chondrocyte implantation with distal realignment (Note: The use of ACI for the patella is considered off-label usage. This procedure was performed with explicit patient informed consent.)

SUBMITTED BY
Tom Minas, MD, and Tim Bryant, RN, Cartilage Repair Center, Brigham and Women's Hospital, Chestnut Hill, Massachusetts, USA

CHIEF COMPLAINT AND HISTORY OF PRESENT ILLNESS

The patient is a 24-year-old man with a history of bilateral recurrent patellar dislocations. He has failed physical therapy measures including taping and bracing to maintain patellofemoral tracking. He has had two prior arthroscopic debridements on both knees, which have been ineffective. He has severe right greater than left anterior knee pain which prevents him from participating in any sporting activities. Stair climbing is painful and requires him to use the handrail to ambulate one step at a time.

PHYSICAL EXAMINATION

Height, 6 ft; weight, 175 lb. Clinical examination reveals a physically fit male with symmetric neutral alignment. He is unable to perform a squat. He has a moderate-sized effusion. Range of motion is symmetric. His quadriceps angle measures 25 degrees with the patella in a reduced position. There is lateral subluxation with quadriceps contraction, and he has profound patellar apprehension. He has moderate patellofemoral crepitus. Meniscal compression testing was unremarkable. His ligament examination is normal.

RADIOGRAPHIC EVALUATION

Plain films were within normal limits, demonstrating normal patellofemoral joint space without subluxation or tilt (Figure C28.1).

SURGICAL INTERVENTION

Arthroscopic evaluation demonstrated grade IV chondrosis involving the central and medial patella. There was obvious subluxation and tilt laterally of the patella with the knee in extension. The trochlea articular surface was normal. A cartilage biopsy for future autologous chondrocyte implantation (ACI) was obtained. Six weeks later, the patient underwent ACI combined with a lateral release, antero-medialization osteotomy (AMZ), and proximal quadriceps advancement. The defect measured 25 mm by 15 mm (Figure C28.2). Postoperatively, the patient was made weight bearing in extension with crutches and began continuous passive motion for 4 to 6 weeks. Activities were gradually advanced as tolerated with impact activities delayed for the first 12 months postoperatively. Radiographs demonstrated healing of his AMZ osteotomy (Figure C28.3).

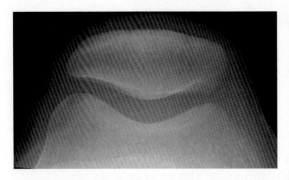

FIGURE C28.1. Preoperative skyline radiograph of the patellofemoral joint demonstrating well-maintained cartilage space.

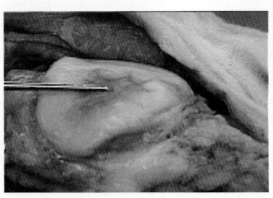

FIGURE C28.2. Appearance of grade IV patellar chondral defect at the time of autologous chondrocyte implantation (ACI).

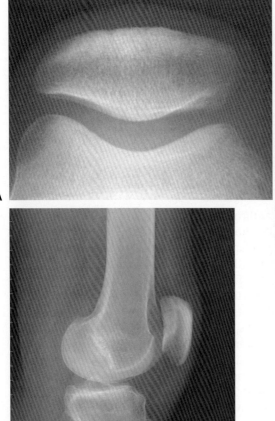

A

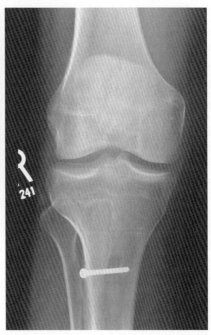

B

C

FIGURE C28.3. Postoperative (A) skyline, (B) anteroposterior, and (C) lateral radiographs demonstrate centralized patella and healed anteromedialization osteotomy.

FOLLOW-UP

One year later, a second-look arthroscopy was performed (Figure C28.4) to remove hardware and to perform a debridement of periosteal overgrowth presenting as retropatellar crepitations with mild discomfort. The patient was painfree afterward, had full range of motion, and ultimately had the other knee reconstructed identically. Four years later he is playing competitive volleyball.

DECISION-MAKING FACTORS

1. Young, active male with symptoms consistent with patellar chondral defect which failed to respond to prior debridements and physical therapy.
2. Contained grade IV defect of the patella of appropriate size for ACI with limited other treatment options other than microfracture (limited goals) and osteochondral allograft (considered not appropriate for a young male with an isolated contained patellar chondral defect).
3. History of patellofemoral instability, increased quadriceps angle, and intraoperative findings of subluxation and tilt leading to decision for AMZ of the tibial tubercle.
4. As apposed to some success in treating inferior and lateral patellar chondral disease with AMZ, it is believed to be less effective when used in isolation for central and medial patellar disease.

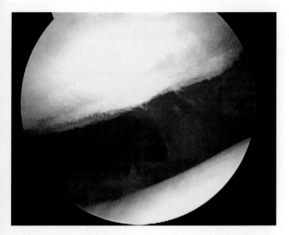

FIGURE C28.4. Arthroscopic appearance of ACI one year after debridement of periosteal overgrowth.

PATHOLOGY
Focal chondral defect medial femoral condyle and varus alignment

TREATMENT
High tibial osteotomy and autologous chondrocyte implantation

SUBMITTED BY
Tom Minas, MD, and Tim Bryant, RN, Cartilage Repair Center, Brigham and
Women's Hospital, Chestnut Hill, Massachusetts, USA

CHIEF COMPLAINT AND HISTORY OF PRESENT ILLNESS

The patient is a 36-year-old man who sustained an injury to the medial femoral condyle of his left knee when he fell from a wave runner directly striking his knee. He developed a large effusion, medial joint pain, difficulty walking, and had catching and giving-way type symptoms. Arthroscopy was performed that demonstrated a large grade IV chondral defect of his medial femoral condyle, which was debrided arthroscopically (Figure C29.1). A second arthroscopic abrasion arthroplasty followed by a period of nonweight bearing also failed to improve his symptoms. Biopsy for future autologous chondrocyte implantation (ACI) was then performed. Physical therapy and antiinflammatory medications were also utilized, leading to no improvement in his symptoms.

PHYSICAL EXAMINATION

Height, 6 ft, 1 in.; weight, 210 lb. At presentation, the patient ambulated with a significant antalgic gait using a cane. Clinical evaluation demonstrated mild varus alignment, quadriceps atrophy, and a small joint effusion. Range of motion was symmetric and full. His medial femoral condyle was tender to palpation, as was his joint line. Meniscal compression testing was unremarkable. His ligament examination was within normal limits.

RADIOGRAPHIC EVALUATION

Plain radiographs demonstrate early medial joint space narrowing compared to the contralateral knee. Long-leg alignment radiographs demonstrated early peripheral medial osteophyte formation, minimal joint space narrowing, and mechanical axis falling into the center of the medial compartment (Figure C29.2).

SURGICAL INTERVENTION

ACI of the medial femoral condyle was performed for a grade IV defect measuring 45 mm long by 8 mm wide (Figure C29.3). A closing-wedge valgus-producing high tibial osteotomy (HTO) of 6 degrees angular correction was also performed to slightly overcorrect the mechani-

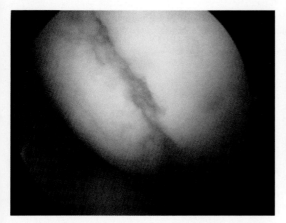

FIGURE C29.1. Arthroscopic appearance of full-thickness chondral defect of medial femoral condyle.

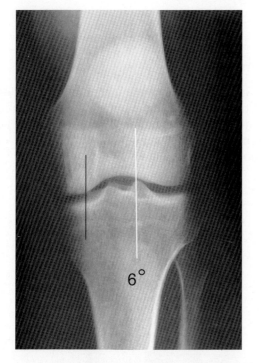

FIGURE C29.2. Cropped standing long-leg alignment radiograph demonstrates the mechanical axis to fall through the center of the medial joint compartment (*black line*) with early medial joint space narrowing compared to the opposite knee (not shown). A planned 6-degree angular correction is drawn (*white line*) to place the mechanical axis through the lateral intercondylar spine in an effort to unload the medial compartment.

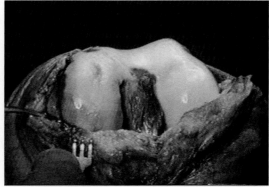

A

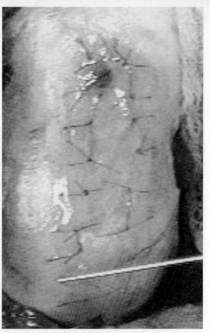

B

FIGURE C29.3. Clinical photographs of the medial femoral condyle at the time of open arthrotomy for autologous chondrocyte implantation (ACI) **(A)**. Note the generalized thinning of the articular cartilage on the medial femoral condyle compared to the lateral femoral condyle and the development of medial peripheral osteophytes compatible with varus alignment and medial compartment overload. These findings were used in part to indicate this patient for simultaneous ACI and high tibial osteotomy (HTO). **(B)** ACI graft being sealed with autologous fibrin glue after injection of autologous cultured chondrocytes.

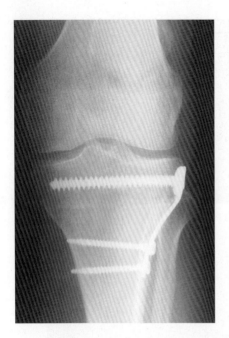

FIGURE C29.4. Standing anteroposterior (AP) radiograph 1 year after reconstructive surgery with restoration of medial joint space.

cal axis to the lateral intercondylar spine (Figure C29.4). Postoperatively, the patient was made nonweight bearing and used continuous passive motion for 6 weeks. Thereafter, he progressed to weight bearing as tolerated. Impact activities were avoided for 12 months postoperatively.

FOLLOW-UP

Within 2 years, the patient returned to sporting activities, hiking, and playing with his children without any symptoms. Five years later he remained symptom free with full range of motion (Figure C29.5).

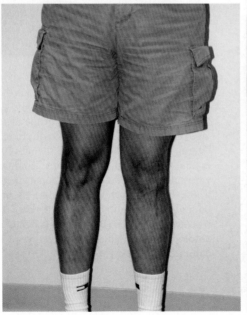
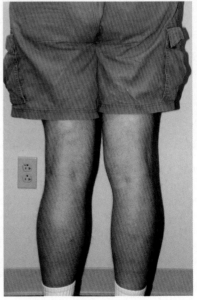

FIGURE C29.5. Clinical appearance of left knee after ACI and HTO demonstrating slight valgus alignment in the **(A)** frontal and **(B)** posterior views.

DECISION-MAKING FACTORS

1. Relatively young male with high physical demand level with symptomatic chondral defect unresponsive to prior treatment attempts.
2. Early joint space narrowing with peripheral osteophyte formation on the medial femoral condyle, and the mechanical axis falling through the center of the medial compartment necessitating both cartilage restoration and unloading osteotomy.
3. General indications for osteotomy included medial compartment disease with slight medial joint space narrowing and mild clinical varus deformity and desire to protect the ACI.
4. ACI chosen over other techniques (osteochondral grafting) because of high level of success demonstrated in lesions of this size and location and the avoidance of creating a subchondral defect.

PATHOLOGY
ACL deficiency with symptomatic trochlear and medial femoral condyle chondral lesions

TREATMENT
ACL reconstruction and autologous chondrocyte implantation

SUBMITTED BY
Brian J. Cole, MD, MBA, Rush Cartilage Restoration Center, Rush University Medical Center, Chicago, Illinois, USA

CHIEF COMPLAINT AND HISTORY OF PRESENT ILLNESS

This patient is a 46-year-old man with complaints of right knee pain, swelling, and giving-way of approximately 2 years duration. He describes a work-related injury occurring 2 years previously when he tripped while carrying a heavy load, sustaining a pop with immediate swelling. Subsequent to that event, he had persistent right knee pain, swelling, and several episodes of his knee giving-way. Following his work-related injury, he underwent right knee arthroscopy, at which time he was diagnosed with at least a partial anterior cruciate ligament (ACL) tear as well as a chondral injury of unclear nature. Chondral debridement was performed without any further treatment. Since that time, he has had severe pain along the medial side of his knee, anterior knee discomfort exacerbated with inclines and declines, recurrent swelling, and giving-way several times a day. Presently, his symptoms are so severe that he is unable to continue working in his present capacity as a manual laborer and presents for evaluation and treatment.

PHYSICAL EXAMINATION

Height, 6ft, 5in.; weight, 214lb. He ambulates with a slightly antalgic gait referable to his right lower extremity. He stands grossly in symmetric neutral alignment. His range of motion is from 0 to 110 degrees as compared to the contralateral side of 0 to 135 degrees. Quadriceps girth on the right side is 2cm smaller than the contralateral normal side. He has a moderate effusion, and his knee is slightly warm to touch. He has moderate tenderness along the medial femoral condyle as well as the medial joint line. He has moderate patellofemoral crepitus with pain on patellar compression. He has no lateral joint line pain. Ligamentous testing reveals a grade II Lachman's examination with no firm endpoint appreciated. Pivot shift testing was difficult secondary to patient guarding.

RADIOGRAPHIC EVALUATION

Forty-five-degree flexion weight-bearing posteroanterior radiographs are unremarkable (Figure C30.1). Long-leg alignment films demonstrate the weight-bearing line to pass

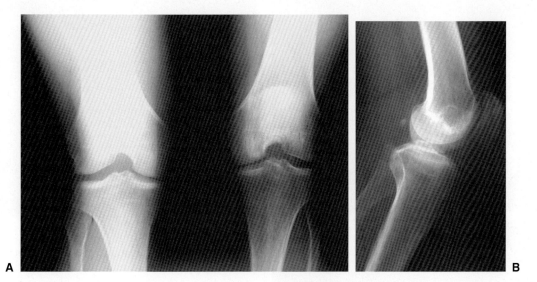

FIGURE C30.1. Forty-five-degree flexion posteroanterior weight-bearing **(A)** and lateral **(B)** radiographs are normal without evidence of joint space narrowing or overt signs of osteoarthritis.

through the center of the knee. Magnetic resonance imaging reveals an articular defect of the medial femoral condyle in the weight-bearing zone as well as some articular thinning of the central trochlea. The ACL appears widened and attenuated on sagittal views.

SURGICAL INTERVENTION

The patient was indicated for arthroscopy to evaluate the articular surfaces as well as the integrity of the ACL. Preoperatively, it was agreed that if the patient had combined pathology of ACL deficiency and articular cartilage disease, that the ACL would be reconstructed at that time using a bone–patellar tendon–bone allograft and, should the articular cartilage disease remain symptomatic, it would be addressed at a later date. It was determined that if the patient had a trochlear lesion that was to be treated with autologous chondrocyte implantation (ACI) then a distal realignment would be be performed concomitantly. Thus, given the magnitude of these individual surgeries and the significant risk for arthrofibrosis if the ACL was initially combined with the ACI, it was decided that the ACL would be reconstructed if indicated during this surgery and the

ACI would be performed with a distal realignment only if symptoms persisted following the ACL reconstruction.

At the time of arthroscopy, the ACL was noted to be deficient. Additionally, two articular defects were noted: a grade IV chondral defect of the trochlea measuring 20 mm by 28 mm and a second grade III to grade IV chondral lesion of the medial femoral condyle measuring 25 mm by 15 mm (Figure C30.2). A 200- to 300-mg specimen of articular cartilage was harvested for culturing from the intercondylar notch during the notchplasty for the ACL reconstruction in anticipation that the ACI would be performed in the future. The ACL was reconstructed without any technical difficulty using the bone–patellar tendon–bone allograft (Figure C30.3). Postoperatively, although the patient did not complain of any further instability, he continued to complain of medial and anterior knee pain with activity-related swelling. At 16 weeks after the ACL reconstruction, the patient underwent ACI of both the trochlear and medial femoral condyle lesions performed in conjunction with a anteromedialization of the tibial tubercle (Figure C30.4). Postoperatively, the patient was initially made nonweight bearing and utilized a continuous passive motion (CPM) machine for

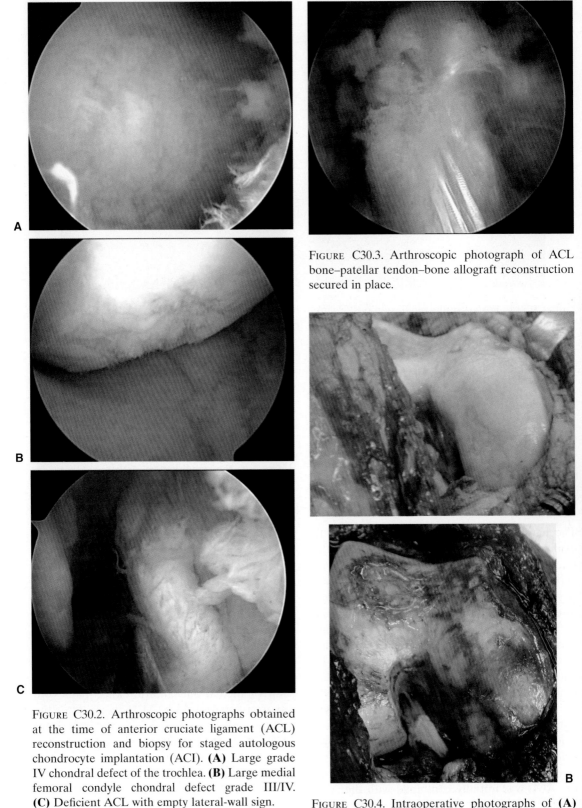

Figure C30.3. Arthroscopic photograph of ACL bone–patellar tendon–bone allograft reconstruction secured in place.

Figure C30.2. Arthroscopic photographs obtained at the time of anterior cruciate ligament (ACL) reconstruction and biopsy for staged autologous chondrocyte implantation (ACI). **(A)** Large grade IV chondral defect of the trochlea. **(B)** Large medial femoral condyle chondral defect grade III/IV. **(C)** Deficient ACL with empty lateral-wall sign.

Figure C30.4. Intraoperative photographs of **(A)** articular cartilage lesions of the trochlea and medial femoral condyle before preparation and **(B)** the same lesions following periosteal patch and fibrin glue placement.

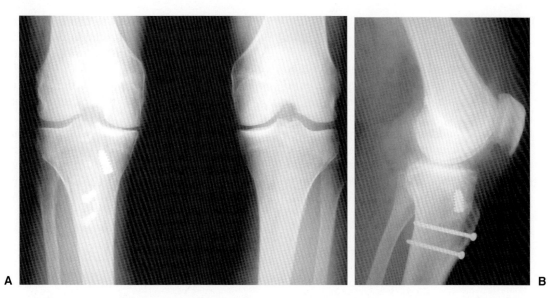

A   B

FIGURE C30.5. Twenty-four-month anteroposterior **(A)** and lateral **(B)** radiographs of the right knee reveal ACL reconstruction and distal realignment osteotomy fixation in satisfactory position.

approximately 6 weeks. Early in the rehabilitation period, his flexion was limited to 45 to 60 degrees to minimize patellofemoral contact forces on the trochlear healing lesion. Patellar mobilization techniques and flexion to 90 degrees were performed daily to prevent stiffness. He was asked to refrain from any impact or ballistic activities for 18 months.

FOLLOW-UP

The patient is now 24 months following ACI and continues to participate in a home exercise program. His subjective complaints mainly focus on some residual difficulty with kneeling and deep squatting. However, he states that he is significantly improved from his preoperative state and that his medial and anterior knee pain has essentially resolved. He denies any residual instability. His range of motion is from 0 to 125 degrees, and he has minimal quadriceps atrophy. His Lachman examination is a grade I with a firm endpoint without a pivot shift. Radiographs reveal a well-healed distal realignment osteotomy and interference screw placement for the ACL graft in a satisfactory position (Figure C30.5). At 24 months, the patient returned for removal of the screws used

to fix the distal realignment and second-look arthroscopy was performed. Both lesions showed excellent fill and integration of hyaline-like cartilage that was minimally fibrillated and relatively firm compared to the surrounding normal articular surfaces (Figure C30.6).

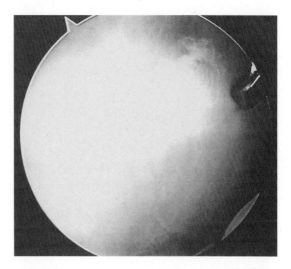

FIGURE C30.6. Twenty-four-month arthroscopic second-look photograph centered on the transition zone between the two defects demonstrates excellent integration and fill following ACI. In this picture, the trochlear defect is visualized almost in its entirety.

DECISION-MAKING FACTORS

1. Complex problem with ligament deficiency in conjunction with multiple symptomatic articular cartilage defects including a trochlear lesion considered less amenable to fresh osteochondral allograft reconstruction.
2. The need to stage the ACL and ACI because (1) some patients with symptoms believed to be related to chondral injury have reduced symptoms following isolated ACL reconstruction and (2) there is significant risk for arthrofibrosis if all procedures (i.e., ACL, ACI, and distal realignment) are performed concomitantly.
3. Failure of prior attempts at articular cartilage debridement and incomplete symptom relief with isolated ACL reconstruction.
4. High-demand individual with multiple articular cartilage lesions considered most amenable to ACI (i.e., due to size and location) as opposed to other options including fresh osteochondral allograft reconstruction.

PATHOLOGY

Focal chondral defect of the medial femoral condyle in a previously menis-
cectomized knee

TREATMENT

Autologous chondrocyte implantation and concomitant medial meniscus allograft transplantation

SUBMITTED BY

Brian J. Cole, MD, MBA, Rush Cartilage Restoration Center, Rush University Medical Center, Chicago, Illinois, USA

CHIEF COMPLAINT AND HISTORY OF PRESENT ILLNESS

This patient is an 18-year-old girl with a chief complaint of persistent medial-sided left knee pain, predominantly weight bearing in nature, and inability to perform any athletic activities. Her history dates back to the age of 15 years when she underwent a medial meniscectomy. Following initial symptom relief, she developed recurrent medial joint line symptoms and activity-related swelling.

PHYSICAL EXAMINATION

Height, 5 ft, 7 in.; weight, 120 lb. She has a normal gait with slight symmetric valgus alignment. Her knee has a small effusion. Her range of motion is normal and symmetric to the contralateral side. She has pain with palpation of her medial femoral condyle and along her medial joint line. Her ligament examination is within normal limits.

RADIOGRAPHIC EVALUATION

Preoperative radiographs obtained for graft sizing demonstrate no significant joint space narrowing and no femoral condyle or tibiofemoral arthritic change (Figure C31.1).

SURGICAL INTERVENTION

At arthroscopy, in addition to evidence of a prior subtotal medial meniscectomy, she was noted to have a concomitant grade IV focal chondral defect of the weight-bearing zone of her medial femoral condyle measuring approximately 15 mm by 18 mm in size (Figure C31.2). An articular cartilage biopsy was harvested from the intercondylar notch, and the patient was indicated for subsequent concomitant medial meniscus allograft transplantation and autologous chondrocyte implantation. Approximately 8 weeks later, a meniscal allograft transplant with bone plugs was performed using an arthroscopically assisted approach (Figure C31.3). Following meniscus repair, a limited medial arthrotomy was made to expose the defect and perform an autologous chondrocyte implantation of the focal chondral defect (Figure C31.4).

Postoperatively, the patient was made non-weight bearing for 4 weeks and used continuous passive motion for 6 weeks for 6 to 8 h/day. Thereafter, she was advanced to weight bearing

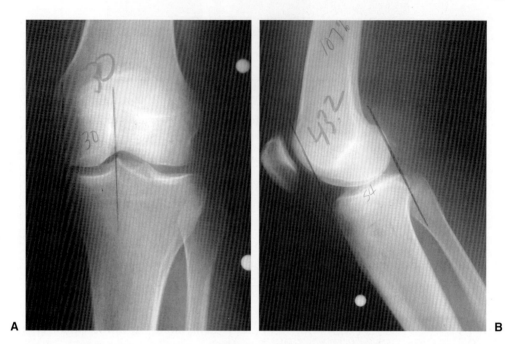

FIGURE C31.1. Anteroposterior **(A)** and lateral **(B)** radiographs demonstrate meniscal sizing with markers in place and no evidence of significant joint space narrowing along the medial tibiofemoral joint.

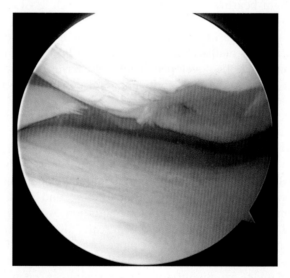

FIGURE C31.2. Arthroscopy demonstrates concomitant pathology of subtotal medial meniscectomy and grade IV focal chondral defect of the medial femoral condyle in the central weight-bearing zone.

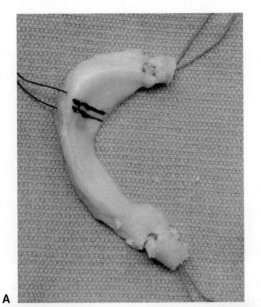

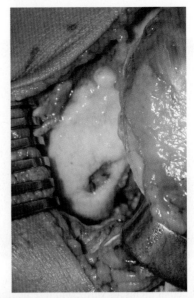

A

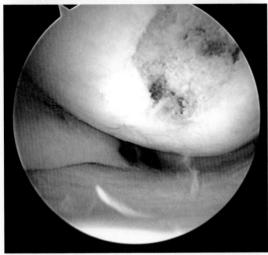

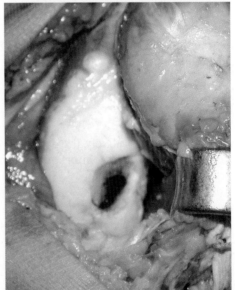

B

FIGURE C31.3. **(A)** Medial meniscus allograft prepared at the time of autologous chondrocyte implantation. **(B)** Meniscus allograft secured in place before performing the arthrotomy and autologous chondrocyte implantation.

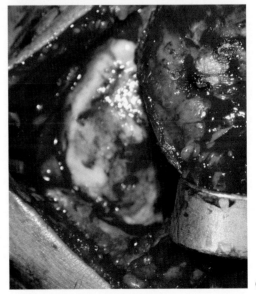

C

FIGURE C31.4. Medial femoral condyle defect before **(A)** and after **(B)** preparation. **(C)** Defect with periosteal patch in place following application of fibrin glue.

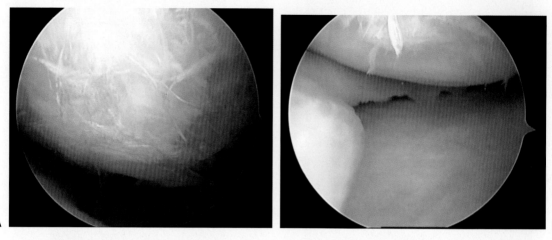

FIGURE C31.5. Twenty-four-month second-look arthroscopy of **(A)** the defect with superficial fibrillation and **(B)** the medial meniscus with complete healing to the periphery and no evidence of shrinkage.

as tolerated. At 12 months, she was permitted to engage in higher-impact activities.

FOLLOW-UP

At 24 months postoperatively, the patient complained of some minor discomfort and activity-related medial joint line pain. A second-look arthroscopy was performed to evaluate the chondral defect and to assess the condition of the medial meniscus (Figure C31.5). The superficial aspect of the autologous chondrocyte implant was gently debrided and the medial meniscus was completely healed to the periphery. At 30 months postoperatively, the patient has returned to all sports with minimal discomfort and denies recurrent effusions or weight-bearing pain.

DECISION-MAKING FACTORS

1. A young, highly active patient with concomitant pathology involving a previous meniscectomy and ipsilateral chondral defect.
2. A relative contraindication to treating either pathology in isolation and the opportunity to treat both abnormalities simultaneously for relative protection of both grafts.
3. Chondral defect size, depth, and location appropriate for autologous chondrocyte implantation with concerns for donor site morbidity and the creation of a subchondral defect if otherwise treated with multiple osteochondral autograft transplants.
4. Rehabilitation tolerant and willingness to be compliant with initial nonweight bearing status.

PATHOLOGY

Focal chondral defect lateral femoral condyle, prior lateral meniscectomy, and small focal chondral defect lateral tibial plateau

TREATMENT

Fresh osteochondral allograft transplant lateral femoral condyle, lateral meniscus transplant, and microfracture lateral tibial plateau

SUBMITTED BY

Brian J. Cole, MD, MBA, Rush Cartilage Restoration Center, Rush University Medical Center, Chicago, Illinois, USA

CHIEF COMPLAINT AND HISTORY OF PRESENT ILLNESS

This patient is a 19-year-old college student who was referred with a chief complaint of right knee weight-bearing lateral-sided knee pain, swelling, and inability to participate in high-level sports. Past surgical history is significant for a right knee lateral meniscectomy performed 5 years before his initial evaluation. The patient did well initially, for 2 years, and then underwent a repeat arthroscopy. At that time, he was documented to have grade III to grade IV changes of the lateral femoral condyle and some early tibial plateau changes. This debridement actually led to some symptom relief until his symptoms recurred, and he presented with progression of pain, swelling, and difficulty playing college-level baseball. At this time, he is unable to play baseball and is having some difficulty with other noncompetitive sports and high-level activities of daily living.

PHYSICAL EXAMINATION

Height, 6 ft, 2 in.; weight, 185 lb. He ambulates with a nonantalgic gait. He stands in symmetric and neutral alignment. His range of motion is 0

to 130 degrees. His right knee has a small effusion. He is tender to palpation over the lateral femoral condyle and lateral joint line. Patellofemoral joint demonstrates good tracking with no evidence of crepitus. Ligamentous testing is within normal limits.

RADIOGRAPHIC EVALUATION

Posteroanterior 45-degree flexion weight-bearing radiograph demonstrates signs of femoral condyle flattening, joint space narrowing along the lateral compartment, and early osteophyte formation along the tibial eminences of the right knee (Figure C32.1).

SURGICAL INTERVENTION

The patient was indicated for a diagnostic arthroscopy, at which time he was noted to have an absent lateral meniscus, a grade III to grade IV lesion of the lateral femoral condyle measuring approximately 30 mm by 30 mm, and an area of nearly grade IV cartilage loss in the central region of the tibial plateau measuring approximately 10 mm by 10 mm (Figure C32.2). A formal microfracture of the lateral tibial plateau

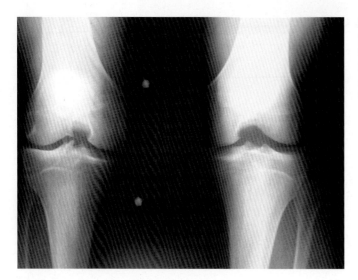

FIGURE C32.1. Forty-five-degree flexion posteroanterior radiograph demonstrates flattening of the right lateral femoral condyle, joint space narrowing, and early degenerative changes along the lateral tibial eminence.

was performed in an effort to prepare the knee for future lateral meniscus transplantation and fresh osteochondral allograft transplantation (Figure C32.3). The patient utilized continuous passive motion postoperatively and was non-weight bearing for approximately 6 weeks.

Six months following the microfracture, the patient still complained of lateral-sided pain, activity-related swelling, and difficulties with

activities of daily living and high-level sports. In consideration of the size of the lateral femoral condyle lesion and the early degenerative changes of the tibia, he was indicated for an osteochondral allograft transplant of the lateral femoral condyle and a simultaneously performed lateral meniscus allograft transplant. Preoperative planning included radiographic sizing images (Figure C32.4). At the time of

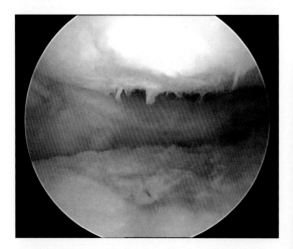

FIGURE C32.2. Index arthroscopy demonstrating diffuse grade IV changes of the lateral femoral condyle, absent lateral meniscus, and a localized area of articular cartilage loss on the lateral tibial plateau measuring approximately 10 mm by 10 mm.

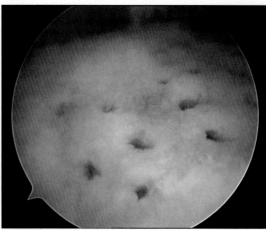

FIGURE C32.3. Focal cartilage defect of the lateral tibial plateau treated with a microfracture technique.

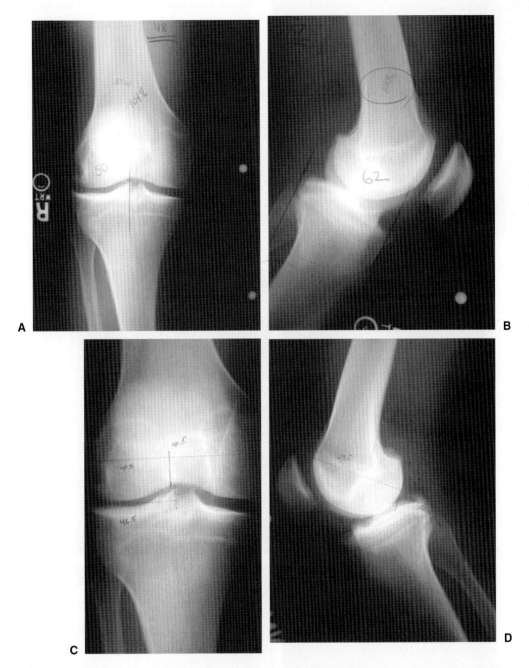

FIGURE C32.4. Anteroposterior **(A)** and lateral **(B)** radiographs with a 100-mm sizing marker in place being utilized for sizing of the allograft meniscus transplant. Anteroposterior **(C)** and lateral **(D)** radiographs with magnification markers to calculate the required fresh osteochondral allograft size.

definitive treatment, the lateral tibial plateau was noted to have excellent fibrocartilage fill of the previously microfractured lesion (Figure C32.5). The patient underwent a fresh osteo- chondral allograft transplant using a 30 mm by 30 mm fresh osteochondral allograft as well as a concomitant lateral meniscus transplant (Figure C32.6).

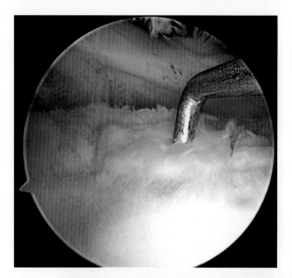

FIGURE C32.5. Six-month second-look arthroscopy following isolated microfracture of the lateral tibial plateau demonstrates fibrocartilage fill of the central tibial plateau defect.

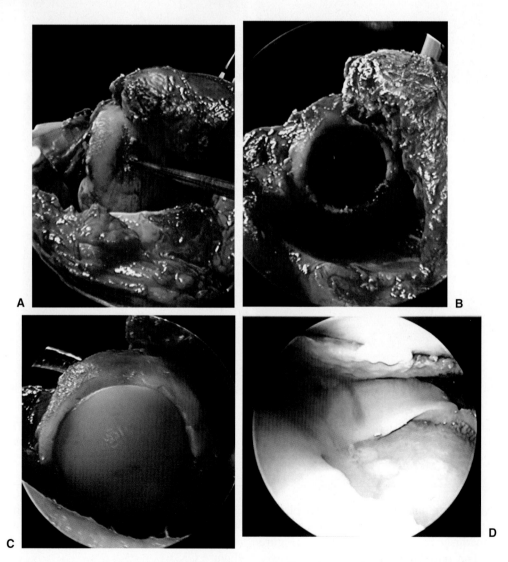

FIGURE C32.6. Intraoperative photograph at the time of arthrotomy of the focal cartilage defect of the lateral femoral condyle **(A)**, with preparing the defect **(B)** for a 30 mm by 30 mm fresh osteochon-dral allograft transplant **(C)**. **(D)** Arthroscopic view of lateral meniscus and osteochondral allograft in place.

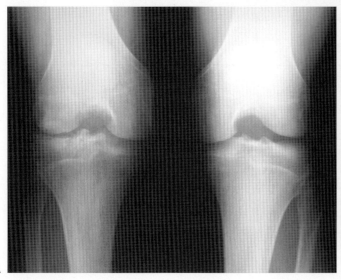
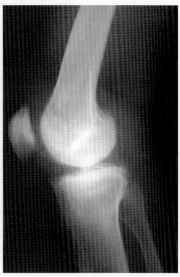

FIGURE C32.7. Eighteen-month postoperative 45-degree flexion weight-bearing posteroanterior **(A)** and lateral **(B)** radiographs demonstrate allograft incorporation, preservation of joint space, incorporation of the lateral meniscus transplant bone bridge, and maintenance of the lateral femoral condyle contour.

FOLLOW-UP

Two years postoperatively, the patient has minimal symptoms and has returned to playing competitive baseball at the collegiate level. Postoperative radiographs demonstrate preservation of the lateral joint space with no progressive joint space loss, as well as incorporation of the osteochondral allograft and of the keyhole bone bridge from the lateral meniscus transplant (Figure C32.7).

DECISION-MAKING FACTORS

1. Relatively young and highly active individual with recurrent symptoms following prior lateral meniscectomy and subsequent debridement and microfracture of the tibial plateau.
2. Microfracture of the tibia given the paucity of other acceptable solutions to treat a relatively small area of grade IV chondral change.
3. Lateral joint line and femoral condyle pain with associated ipsilateral meniscal deficiency and articular cartilage disease.
4. Large defect of the femoral condyle with early degenerative change of the opposing tibial plateau considered more tolerant of a fresh osteochondral allograft than autologous chondrocyte implantation.

PATHOLOGY

Bipolar focal chondral defects of the patellofemoral joint with patellar instability

TREATMENT

Autologous chondrocyte implantation of the patella and trochlea with distal realignment (Note that the use of ACI for the patella or for bipolar defects is considered off-label usage, but was indicated and performed with explicit patient and family informed consent and under the guidance of an Institutional Review Board protocol allowing prospective study of this patient at the author's institution.)

SUBMITTED BY

Brian J. Cole, MD, MBA, Rush Cartilage Restoration Center, Rush University Medical Center, Chicago, Illinois, USA

CHIEF COMPLAINT AND HISTORY OF PRESENT ILLNESS

This patient is an 18-year-old female whose chief complaint is that of persistent anterior knee pain, swelling, and recurrent patellar instability. As an adolescent, the patient had persistent anterior knee pain and recurrent subluxation of the patella. She underwent a lateral release at the age of 12, but continued to do poorly until her early teenage years. Subsequent to this, she came to arthroscopy and was diagnosed with a focal chondral defect of the patella and trochlea; the patella was debrided and the trochlea was treated with abrasion arthroplasty. Despite this treatment, the patient continued to have persistent instability and activity-related swelling and anterior knee pain. She was subsequently referred for cartilage restoration 3 years after her last surgery.

PHYSICAL EXAMINATION

Height, 5 ft, 6 in.; weight, 140 lb. The patient ambulates with a nonantalgic gait. She stands in approximately 4 degrees of physiologic valgus bilaterally. Her Q angle measures 10 degrees. Her range of motion is symmetric from 5 degrees of hyperextension to 130 degrees of flexion. She demonstrates some hypermobility of her other joints, including elbow hyperextension and metacarpophalangeal hyperextension. She demonstrates patellofemoral apprehension, a moderate effusion of her left knee, three-quadrant translation laterally, and one-quadrant translation medially of the patella with the knee in extension. She has a palpable clunk at 40 degrees of flexion during active range of motion assessment. Her medial and lateral joint lines are not painful. Her ligament examination is within normal limits.

RADIOGRAPHIC EVALUATION

At presentation, her radiographs demonstrated no evidence of overt patellofemoral arthritis or cystic change. The lateral radiograph demonstrated some evidence of patella alta. The computed tomography (CT) scan demonstrated lateral displacement of the patella relative to the trochlea and mild trochlear hypoplasia. There was no evidence of involve-

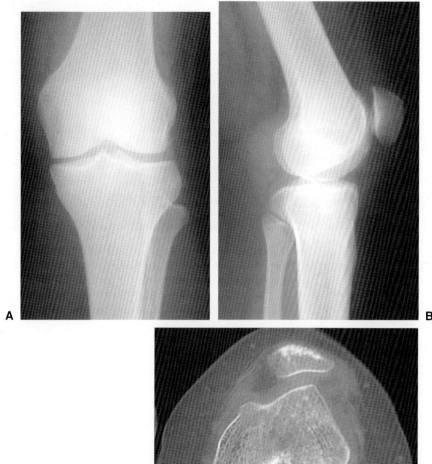

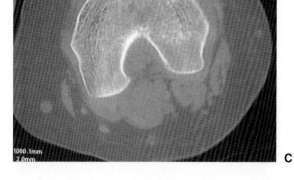

FIGURE C33.1. Anteroposterior **(A)** and lateral **(B)** radiographs demonstrate no evidence of overt patellofemoral arthritis. Lateral radiograph demonstrates patella alta. **(C)** Axial CT scan of the patellofemoral joint demonstrates some lateral displacement of the patella relative to the trochlea and mild trochlear hypoplasia.

ment of the patellar subchondral bone (Figure C33.1).

SURGICAL INTERVENTION

At the time of arthroscopic biopsy for autologous chondrocyte implantation (ACI), a 12 mm by 14 mm grade IV focal chondral defect of the central-to-lateral aspect of the patella and a 12 mm by 14 mm focal chondral defect of the trochlea with fibrocartilaginous fill were identified (Figure C33.2). A biopsy was obtained from the intercondylar notch, and subsequent to this the patient underwent ACI of her bipolar defects of the patella and trochlea about 8 weeks later (Figure C33.3). At the same time, a very oblique anteromedializa-

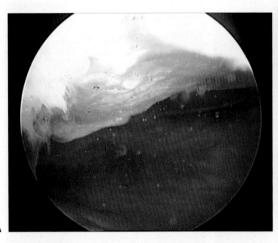
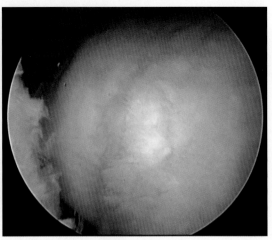
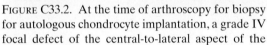

FIGURE C33.2. At the time of arthroscopy for biopsy for autologous chondrocyte implantation, a grade IV focal defect of the central-to-lateral aspect of the patella **(A)** and a focal defect of the trochlea with fibrocartilaginous fill **(B)** are identified.

tion of the tibial tubercle was performed. Postoperative radiographs demonstrate elevation and translation of the tibial tubercle (Figure C33.4).

Postoperatively, she was made heel-touch weight bearing for approximately 6 weeks until radiographs demonstrated evidence of healing of the distal realignment. Although she was allowed to flex her knee daily to 90 degrees, continuous passive motion was restricted to 45 to 60 degrees of flexion during its use for the first 6 postoperative weeks. She advanced through the traditional rehabilitation protocol for ACI of the patellofemoral joint. She was

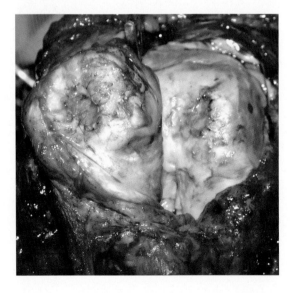

FIGURE C33.3. Intraoperative photograph of autologous chondrocyte implantation for bipolar defects of the patella and trochlea.

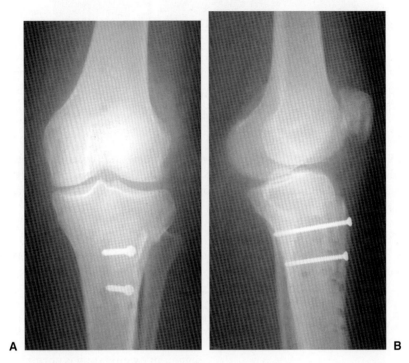

FIGURE C33.4. Postoperative anteroposterior **(A)** and lateral **(B)** radiographs demonstrate elevation and translation of the tibial tubercle.

asked to refrain from any impact or ballistic activities for 18 months.

FOLLOW-UP

At early follow-up at approximately 18 months, the patient has significantly less pain, no recurrent patellar instability, and she is resuming low levels of activities such as biking, hiking, swimming, and the stair machine for her daily exercise regimen. Postoperative radiographs demonstrate elevation and translation of the tibial tubercle with no evidence of patellofemoral arthritic change (Figure C33.4).

DECISION-MAKING FACTORS

1. Young, highly symptomatic patient with failed primary attempt to achieve cartilage repair tissue of the patellofemoral joint.
2. Bipolar defect of the patellofemoral joint with no other treatment options other than, possibly, osteochondral allograft.
3. Recurrent patellar instability in addition to patellar defect likely to benefit from antero-medialization procedure.
4. Expected additional marginal benefit from concomitant resurfacing procedure in addition to anteromedialization.

PATHOLOGY
Bipolar focal chondral defects of the patellofemoral joint

TREATMENT
Autologous chondrocyte implantation of the patella and trochlea (Note that the use of ACI for the patella or for bipolar defects is considered off-label usage, but was indicated and performed with explicit patient informed consent.)

SUBMITTED BY
Jack Farr, MD, Cartilage Restoration Center of Indiana, OrthoIndy, Indianapolis, Indiana, USA

CHIEF COMPLAINT AND HISTORY OF PRESENT ILLNESS

The patient is a 28-year-old man who works in his family boiler company as an estimator/troubleshooter. He has a long history of bilateral patellofemoral pain, right worse than left. In his late teens he enjoyed basketball, but had to stop all sports because of severe anterior knee pain and limited his activities to level-ground walking. Review of the operative record reveals that 4 years before presentation, at age 24, he underwent a lateral release and anteromedialization (AMZ) procedure, which was performed with a steep slope osteotomy as malalignment was mild. The articular surfaces at that time were intact, except at the patellofemoral joint where contained grade III chondral defects were noted on the patella and trochlea, each measuring 2 cm by 2 cm. These lesions were treated with mechanical chondroplasty at the time of the AMZ. The patient had minimal symptoms until 2 years later when symptoms similar to his condition 4 years ago developed.

PHYSICAL EXAMINATION

Height, 6 ft, 10 in.; weight, 280 lb. Level-ground gait is normal. Mild symmetric valgus alignment is present. He has a well-healed incision from his prior AMZ. His range of motion is symmetric from 0 to 135 degrees of flexion. His ligament examination is normal. Patellar apprehension is absent. Tenderness is isolated to the patellofemoral joint, where there is 1 cm of medial and lateral displacement. Tilt is reversible to neutral.

RADIOGRAPHIC EVALUATION

Preoperative radiographs of his right knee reveal maintenance of tibiofemoral joint space with near-neutral alignment. Merchant view shows joint space maintenance and a central patella. Evidence of a prior AMZ with internal fixation is present (Figure C34.1).

SURGICAL INTERVENTION

Right knee arthroscopy revealed progression in the size and grade (to grade IV) of the chondral defects of both the patella and trochlea. The trochlea had an intralesional osteophyte treated with impaction (Figure C34.2). Cartilage biopsy was performed. Six weeks later, autologous chondrocyte implantation (ACI)

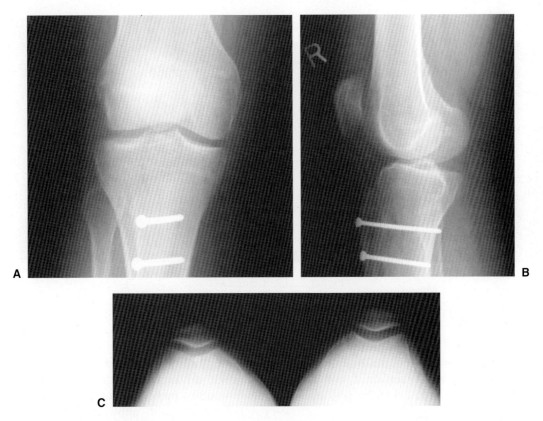

FIGURE C34.1. Radiographs after initial anteromedialization (AMZ) osteotomy. Anteroposterior **(A)**, lateral **(B)**, and Merchant **(C)** views show maintenance of joint space and central patella.

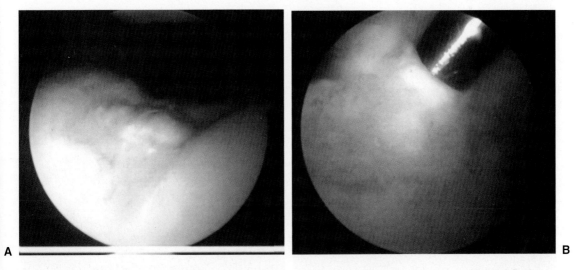

FIGURE C34.2. Intralesional trochlear osteophyte **(A)**, raised appearance **(B)**, impaction **(C)**, and flush area of prior osteophyte **(D)**.

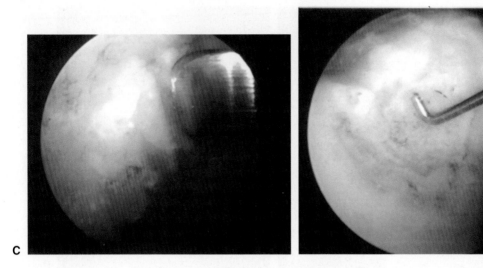

C   D

FIGURE C34.2. *Continued*

was performed on the patella and trochlear lesions, both of which remained contained, grade IV, and measured 2.5 cm by 3 cm at each site (Figure C34.3).

Although he was allowed to flex his knee daily to 90 degrees, continuous passive motion was restricted to 45 to 60 degrees of flexion during its use for the first 4 postoperative weeks. He advanced through the traditional rehabilitation protocol for ACI of the patellofemoral joint allowing early weight bearing in extension. He was asked to refrain from any impact or ballistic activities for 18 months.

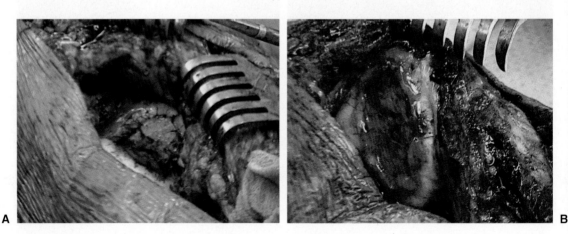

A   B

FIGURE C34.3. Intraoperative autologous chondrocyte implantation (ACI) patches in place in the **(A)** trochlea and **(B)** patella.

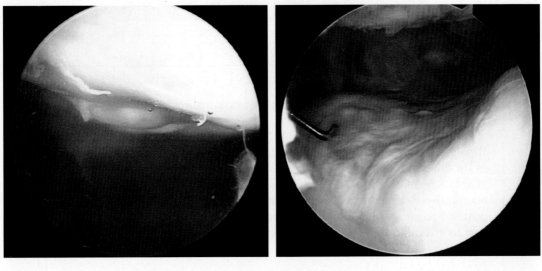

FIGURE C34.4. Second-look arthroscopic view of ACI filling both the **(A)** patellar and **(B)** trochlear defects.

FOLLOW-UP

Postoperatively the patient had progressive diminution of pain. After his pain resolved, he slipped in mud and had acute, new onset medial joint line pain. The medial pain persisted and he was subsequently evaluated arthroscopically. Arthroscopy revealed the areas of ACI were filling with full peripheral integration (Figure C34.4). The medial pain resolved with debridement of impinging scar. At present he is without pain during activities of daily living, and his contralateral patellofemoral pain is now his main concern.

DECISION-MAKING FACTORS

1. Young, highly symptomatic patient with failed primary attempt to unload his patellofemoral joint.
2. Bipolar defect of the patellofemoral joint with no other treatment options other than possibly osteochondral allograft.
3. Bipolar contained lesions treated initially with AMZ in an effort to mechanically unload the defects.
4. Impaction of intralesional osteophyte preceding ACI versus burring at time of ACI in an effort to minimize bleeding.

PATHOLOGY

Lateral compartment tibiofemoral degenerative arthrosis

TREATMENT

Bipolar fresh osteochondral allograft transplant (At this juncture, the author, as do other surgeons who perform osteochondral allograft transplantation, assigns a significantly guarded prognosis to bipolar biologic resurfacing operations. These surgeons obtain full patient informed consent regarding the guarded prognosis and proceed with surgery only under the auspice that revision to arthroplasty is not knowingly compromised should the allograft fail.)

SUBMITTED BY

Jack Farr, MD, Cartilage Restoration Center of Indiana, OrthoIndy, Indianapolis, Indiana, USA

CHIEF COMPLAINT AND HISTORY OF PRESENT ILLNESS

This patient is a 38-year-old male construction supervisor who is referred for consideration of autologous chondrocyte implantation (ACI) to treat persistently symptomatic chondrosis of the left knee at the site of an old lateral compartment injury. His pain has gradually increased to the point where he can only walk short distances with a cane and an unloader brace. He is on partial disability as he can only perform sitting duties at work. Review of his history revealed a distant sports injury, which was treated with arthroscopic partial lateral meniscectomy. His pain gradually recurred, and he underwent another arthroscopy where a lateral femoral condyle grade IV chondral lesion measuring 2.5 cm by 2.5 cm was treated with abrasion arthroplasty. Additional lateral meniscus was also removed. The tibial plateau was intact at that time. The patient was evaluated for cartilage restoration options and elected to proceed with staging arthroscopy and probable harvest of biopsy for ACI. Insur-

ance appeals delayed staging surgery for 1.5 years.

PHYSICAL EXAMINATION

Height, 5 ft, 10 in.; weight, 165 lb. Gait on the left is severely antalgic even with use of a cane and unloader brace. No effusion is noted. Clinical alignment is in neutral. Range of motion demonstrates 5 degrees of flexion loss compared to the contralateral knee. His ligament examination is normal. Pain is isolated to the lateral joint line without mechanical symptoms. Patellar tracking is normal.

RADIOGRAPHIC EVALUATION

Marked lateral joint space narrowing is noted on 45-degree posteroanterior weight-bearing radiographs. Only mild joint space narrowing is noted on anteroposterior films, and no osteophytes are noted. Alignment is 2 degrees of varus.

FIGURE C35.1. Intraoperative photograph demonstrates exposed bone of the distal lateral femoral condyle and absent lateral meniscus.

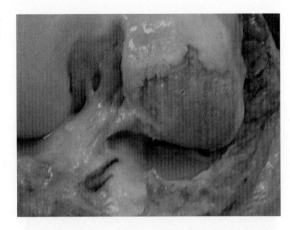

SURGICAL INTERVENTION

At arthroscopy, there was new extensive involvement of the tibial plateau with exposed bone without lateral or posterior containment. Evidence of a complete prior lateral meniscectomy was present. The lateral femoral condyle had exposed bone evident with knee flexion past 90 degrees (Figure C35.1). ACI biopsy was not performed in light of the extensive nature of the chondrosis, uncontained lesions, and progression to bipolar status. At the time of definitive treatment, the arthritic regions of the distal femoral condyle and proximal tibial plateau were osteotomized in preparation for fresh osteochondral allograft transplantation.

The surgical exposure was facilitated by tibial tubercle osteotomy and osteotomy of the femoral insertion of the lateral collateral ligament and popliteus tendon as well as Gerdy's tubercle (Figure C35.2). Fresh osteochondral shell allografts were prepared and implanted. These grafts included the lateral femoral condyle and lateral tibial plateau with the attached lateral meniscus (Figure C35.3).

Postoperatively, the patient was made non-weight bearing for 8 weeks. Continuous passive motion was used immediately with early efforts to regain full range of motion. Any consideration for high-impact activities was delayed for 18 months.

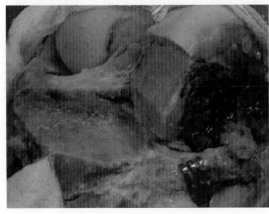

FIGURE C35.2. Host prepared with minimal bone resection of the distal femoral condyle and proximal tibial plateau. Note osteotomized origin of the lateral collateral ligament and popliteus tendon.

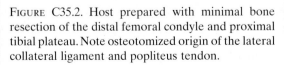

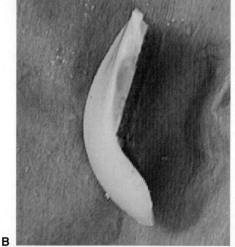

A

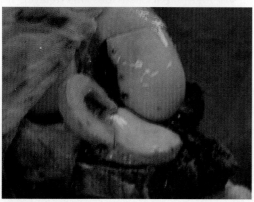

B

FOLLOW-UP

Eight-week postoperative radiographs revealed initial graft incorporation and maintenance of joint spaces (Figure C35.4). At 8 months, the patient regained full motion and is ambulating without an aid and without pain.

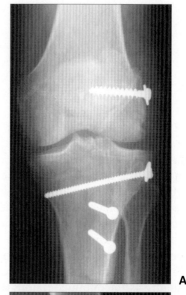

A

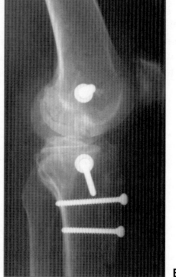

B

FIGURE C35.3. Fresh lateral femoral condyle osteochondral allograft before **(A)** and after **(B)** preparation. **(C)** Distal lateral femoral condyle and composite tibial plateau allograft in place fixed with cortical bone pins.

FIGURE C35.4. Postoperative anteroposterior **(A)** and lateral **(B)** radiographs. Note cortical bone pins and fixation of osteotomized lateral epicondyle, Gerdy's tubercle, and tibial tubercle fragment.

DECISION-MAKING FACTORS

1. Relatively young, but severely symptomatic individual with unicompartmental pathology.
2. Young age as a relative contraindication to arthroplasty (i.e., unicompartmental or total knee arthroplasty).
3. Bipolar disease with large uncontained lesions as a relative contraindication to ACI.
4. Neutral to varus alignment eliminating distal femoral osteotomy as a legitimate solution.
5. Absent lateral meniscus in addition to degenerative tibial plateau requiring replacement with composite meniscus and osteoarticular graft.

PATHOLOGY
Isolated patellofemoral arthritis

TREATMENT
Bipolar patellofemoral fresh osteochondral allograft with distal realignment
(At this juncture, the author, as do other surgeons who perform osteochondral allograft transplantation, assigns a significantly guarded prognosis to bipolar biologic resurfacing operations. These surgeons obtain full patient informed consent regarding the guarded prognosis and proceed with surgery only under the auspice that revision to arthroplasty is not knowingly compromised should the allograft fail.)

SUBMITTED BY
Jack Farr, MD, Cartilage Restoration Center of Indiana, OrthoIndy, Indianapolis, Indiana, USA

CHIEF COMPLAINT AND HISTORY OF PRESENT ILLNESS

This patient is a 37-year-old female nurse who presented with progressive patellofemoral pain of her right knee. She had intermittent pain since a medial arthrotomy was performed 22 years previously to treat a "crushed" patella she sustained from direct impact. Her pain increases with any increase in activity. She experiences marked pain at the end of an 8-hour nursing shift. She is unable to perform squats or climb stairs. Repeated attempts at rehabilitation failed to reduce her symptoms.

PHYSICAL EXAMINATION

Height, 5ft, 5in.; weight, 135lb; body mass index of 23. She ambulates with an antalgic gait. Limb alignment is neutral. She is unable to step up on a 6-in. step secondary to pain. Range of motion is from 5 to 130 degrees of flexion. Pain and crepitus are limited to the patellofemoral joint. She has no patellar appre-

hension. Her ligament examination is normal. Meniscal findings are absent. Quadriceps bulk is near normal.

RADIOGRAPHIC EVALUATION

Posteroanterior 45-degree flexion weight-bearing radiographs demonstrate neutral alignment with no joint space narrowing. Merchant views demonstrate patellofemoral arthritis in the right knee with no significant subluxation or tilt (Figure C36.1), but there is joint space narrowing at the medial aspect of the patellofemoral articulation.

SURGICAL INTERVENTION

At the staging arthroscopy, the entire trochlea had grade III and IV change and the medial 60% of the patella had grade III–IV change. Both the lesions were diffuse and incompletely contained (Figure C36.2). The tibiofemoral joint was normal. The patient then underwent patellofemoral resurfacing with fresh osteo-

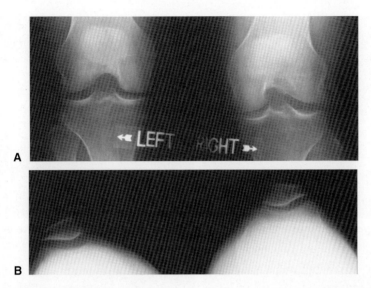

FIGURE C36.1. Preoperative posteroanterior 45-degree flexion weight-bearing **(A)** and Merchant **(B)** radiographs demonstrate isolated patellofemoral arthritis with significant joint space narrowing of the right knee.

chondral shell allografts (Figure C36.3). Milled cortical allograft bone pins were used for fixation. The exposure was through a steep anteromedialization of the tibial tubercle, which allowed the patella to remain central while the tubercle was elevated in an attempt to potentially decrease the load on the allograft shells.

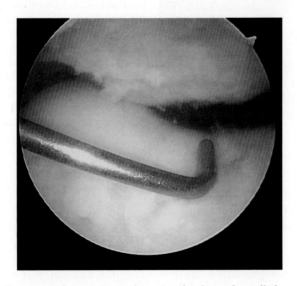

FIGURE C36.2. Staging arthroscopy demonstrates the extensive loss of patellofemoral articular cartilage.

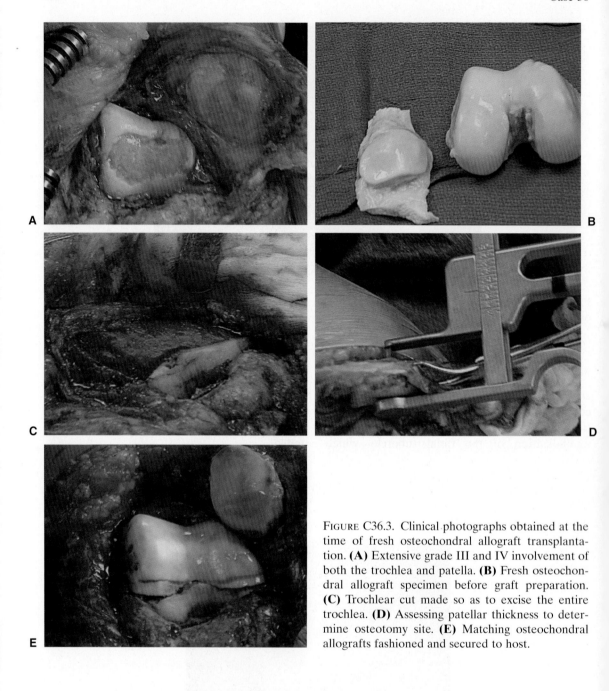

FIGURE C36.3. Clinical photographs obtained at the time of fresh osteochondral allograft transplantation. **(A)** Extensive grade III and IV involvement of both the trochlea and patella. **(B)** Fresh osteochondral allograft specimen before graft preparation. **(C)** Trochlear cut made so as to excise the entire trochlea. **(D)** Assessing patellar thickness to determine osteotomy site. **(E)** Matching osteochondral allografts fashioned and secured to host.

Postoperatively, the patient was made weight bearing as tolerated with two crutches using a hinged brace set at 0 to 30 degrees for protection. Continuous passive motion was used for 3 weeks, with early full range of motion allowed immediately as tolerated. Return to unrestricted activities was permitted after 6 months.

FOLLOW-UP

The patient is nearly symptom free with maintenance of transplant position and joint space (Figure C36.4). She has minimal patellofemoral crepitus, and range of motion is comparable to her preoperative evaluation.

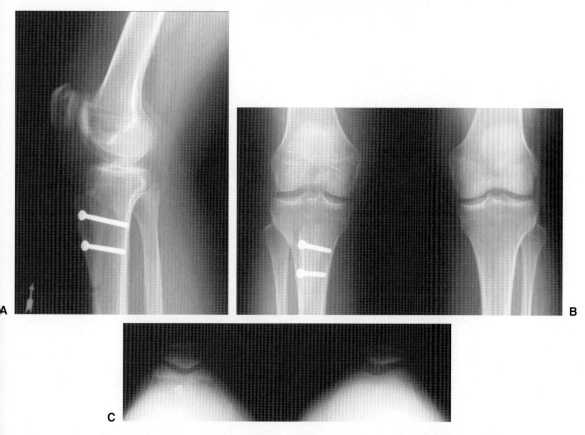

FIGURE C36.4. Postoperative radiographs obtained within the first 3 months after surgery. Lateral **(A)**, anteroposterior weight-bearing **(B)**, and Merchant **(C)** views demonstrate anatomic placement of the graft with cortical bone dowels in place without evidence of graft collapse or dislodgement.

DECISION-MAKING FACTORS

1. Relatively young, active individual with specific symptoms related to isolated posttraumatic patellofemoral osteoarthritis.
2. Young age as a relative contraindication to arthroplasty (i.e., patellofemoral or total knee arthroplasty).
3. Bipolar defects that are large, diffuse, and incompletely contained, virtually eliminating other cartilage restoration procedures as viable options.
4. Unloading considerations as a part of patellofemoral cartilage restoration include a steep oblique anteromedialization to protect and unload the healing grafts.

PATHOLOGY

Posttraumatic medial femoral condyle defect, varus instability, and deformity with significant motion loss

TREATMENT

Open release, staged fresh osteochondral allograft transplantation with medial opening-wedge high tibial osteotomy followed by lateral collateral ligament reconstruction

SUBMITTED BY

Brian J. Cole, MD, MBA, Rush Cartilage Restoration Center, Rush University Medical Center, Chicago, Illinois, USA

CHIEF COMPLAINT AND HISTORY OF PRESENT ILLNESS

The patient is a 26-year-old man who sustained a high-energy injury to the lateral aspect of his right knee when a tree trunk struck him while he was working as a tree trimmer. This injury was documented as a lateral-sided ligament injury with an intraarticular fracture of the medial femoral condyle. Initial treatment included open reduction and internal fixation of a medial femoral condyle fracture. Postoperatively, he was made nonweight bearing and his knee was immobilized for several weeks, leading to significant motion loss. At his initial presentation 6 months following this operation, he complained of significant knee stiffness, instability, and medial-sided right knee pain.

PHYSICAL EXAMINATION

Height. 5 ft, 6 in.; weight, 150 lb. Examination of the right knee reveals significant varus alignment with a flexed-knee antalgic gait accompanied by a lateral thrust (e.g., triple varus thrust) (Figure C37.1). His incisions are well healed without any signs of infection. He has a 20-degree flexion contracture and cannot flex past 90 degrees. His patellar mobility is severely limited. He has significant medial joint line and femoral condyle tenderness. On stress testing, he has grade 2 varus instability with an end-point, and minimal increases in external rotation at 30 and 90 degrees of flexion compared to the contralateral side. His reverse pivot shift and posterior drawer tests are negative. His anterior cruciate ligament (ACL) examination is normal. He is neurovascularly intact distally.

RADIOGRAPHIC EVALUATION

Initial radiographs obtained 6 months following his open reduction demonstrated limited internal fixation of his medial femoral condyle fracture with a significant defect remaining along the central weight-bearing zone (Figure C37.2). Long-leg alignment views obtained following hardware removal and open release of adhesions demonstrated a varus deformity measuring 12 degrees of mechanical axis varus (Figure C37.3).

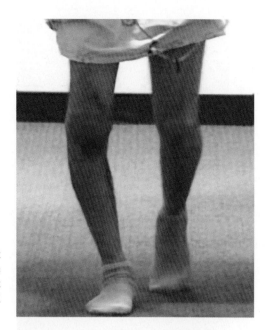

Figure C37.1. Clinical photograph obtained during gait demonstrates significant dynamic varus thrust of the patient's right knee due to lateral collateral ligament insufficiency and osteochondral defect of the medial femoral condyle.

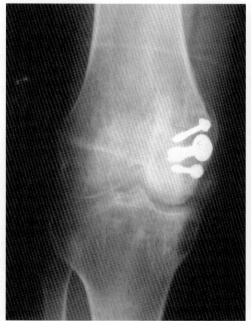

A

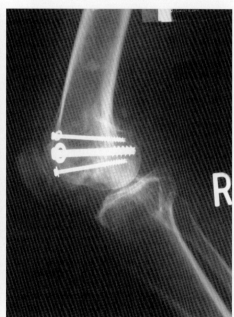

B

Figure C37.2. Anteroposterior **(A)** and lateral **(B)** radiographs obtained 6 months after open reduction and internal fixation of the medial femoral condyle fracture demonstrate residual osteochondral defect along the weight-bearing aspect of the medial femoral condyle. Also noted is significant osteopenia resulting from a prolonged period of protected weight bearing.

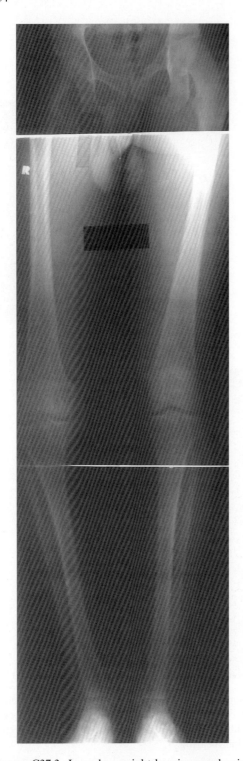

SURGICAL INTERVENTION

Three issues were particularly concerning in this patient: motion loss, varus instability, and a posttraumatic defect of his medial femoral condyle. Initially, the principal focus was on helping the patient regain a functional range of motion. Because of the significant periarticular scarring, the patient underwent his second surgical procedure, which included an arthrotomy, removal of his hardware, extensive intraarticular release, manipulation under anesthesia, and placement in a well-padded long-leg hyperextension cast. Evaluation of his articular surfaces (Figure C37.4) demonstrated a large medial femoral condyle defect measuring 30 mm by 30 mm with more than 10 mm of subchondral bone loss. Following cast removal at 3 days, the patient was placed in an aggressive physical therapy program.

Four months following his open release, his flexion contracture was reduced to 5 degrees and he obtained nearly 120 degrees of flexion. He continued to complain of significant medial knee pain and varus instability. At that time he was indicated for an opening-wedge high tibial osteotomy and fresh osteochondral allograft

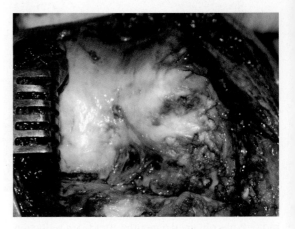

FIGURE C37.4. Intraoperative photograph obtained during the arthrotomy, lysis of adhesions, and hardware removal which was required to regain functional range of motion and prepare for future reconstruction procedures. Note the significant osteochondral defect of the medial femoral condyle measuring approximately 30 mm by 30 mm.

FIGURE C37.3. Long-leg weight-bearing mechanical axis radiograph obtained following arthrotomy and hardware removal. Note the significant static varus deformity of the right knee due to the lateral collateral ligament insufficiency and osteochondral defect of the medial femoral condyle.

transplant of his medial femoral condyle. Any attempts to reconstruct his lateral collateral ligament were delayed because of the possibility that the osteotomy might reduce or eliminate his complaints of varus instability and because of the significant risk of recurrent stiffness following the necessary rehabilitation and protection required of this procedure.

Thus, his third surgery, occurring approximately 1 year after his initial injury, included a 15-degree opening-wedge medial high tibial osteotomy with an iliac crest bone graft and a 30mm by 30mm fresh osteochondral shell allograft transplant (Figure C37.5). A headless cannulated compression screw was used to supplement the press-fit fixation of the osteochondral graft.

His knee pain and motion continued to improve over the ensuing 6 months and, despite radiographic evidence of healing at the osteotomy site with valgus alignment (Figure C37.6), he continued to complain of some varus instability, albeit significantly less than his

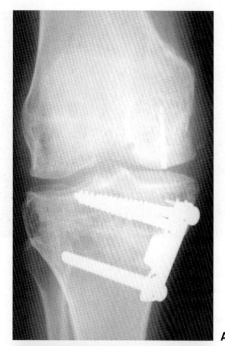

A

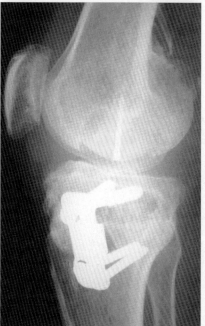

B

FIGURE C37.6. Anteroposterior **(A)** and lateral **(B)** radiographs obtained 6 months after fresh osteochondral allograft transplantation of the medial femoral condyle and medial opening-wedge high tibial osteotomy. Note evidence of graft integration without evidence of collapse and bony union at the osteotomy site.

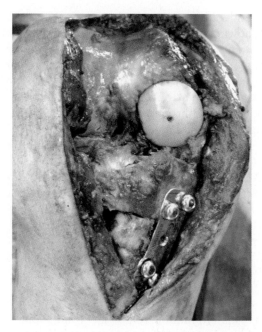

FIGURE C37.5. Intraoperative photograph obtained following placement of the fresh osteochondral allograft and completion of the medial opening-wedge high tibial osteotomy. Note the tricortical iliac crest bone autograft positioned within the osteotomy site.

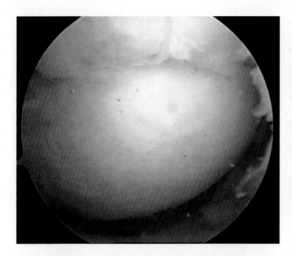

FIGURE C37.7. Arthroscopic view of the medial femoral condyle obtained 7 months following osteochondral allograft transplantation. Note the lack of any articular degeneration of the allograft transplant.

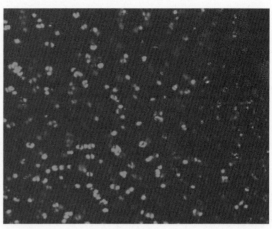

FIGURE C37.9. Biopsy obtained at second-look arthroscopy. Live/dead cell technique analyzed using confocal light microscopy demonstrates a large number of living donor chondrocytes (*green cells*) with minimal evidence of cell death (*red cells*) and maintenance of the cartilage architecture. 10× original magnification. (Courtesy of James M. Williams, PhD, Rush University)

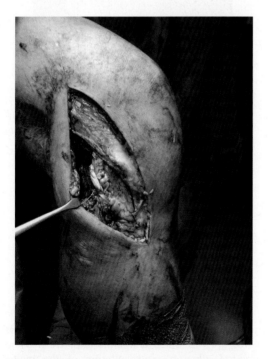

FIGURE C37.8. Intraoperative photograph of the lateral collateral ligament reconstruction using a hamstring allograft. Note graft fixed at isometric point of femur and through a drill hole in the proximal fibula with bioabsorbable screw placed within the fibular tunnel.

preoperative level of instability. Seven months following the transplant and osteotomy, the patient underwent second-look arthroscopy (Figure C37.7) and a lateral ligament reconstruction using a hamstring allograft fixed at the isometric point of the lateral femoral condyle and passed through the proximal fibula in a figure-of-eight configuration (Figure C37.8). A 1-mm biopsy of the fresh osteochondral allograft was obtained at that time (Figure C37.9). Postoperatively, the patient was made protected weight bearing in an extension brace for the first 6 weeks and progressed to weight bearing and activities as tolerated over the ensuing 6 months.

FOLLOW-UP

At his 18-month follow-up evaluation, he achieved nearly full extension with 120 degrees of flexion. His knee was stable to varus stress in extension and various degrees of flexion. He continues to have a slightly antalgic gait, but complains of no pain along the medial side of his knee. Although he states he is significantly improved compared to the results following his open reduction and internal fixation, he feels he is not yet able to return to work where climbing and squatting would be required. He continues to participate in an aggressive home exercise program.

DECISION-MAKING FACTORS

1. High-energy injury young, active, male laborer resulting in significant osteochondral defect and varus instability.
2. A requirement to restore motion before articular reconstruction.
3. Large osteochondral defect requiring structural support considered less amenable to other cartilage restoration techniques.
4. Varus alignment requiring medial high tibial osteotomy to correct the deformity, protect the cartilage allograft, and potentially eliminate symptoms of varus instability.
5. Delayed reconstruction of the lateral collateral ligament due to the opposing early-phase rehabilitation compared to the early and full range of motion required following osteochondral allograft transplantation. In addition, the potential for eliminating the need for ligament reconstruction altogether because of the corrective effects of the opening-wedge high tibial osteotomy.

PATHOLOGY
Chondral defects with prior medial and lateral meniscectomy and varus alignment

TREATMENT
Staged high tibial osteotomy followed by single-stage autologous chondrocyte implantation and medial and lateral meniscus allograft transplantation

SUBMITTED BY
Jack Farr, MD, Cartilage Restoration Center of Indiana, OrthoIndy, Indianapolis, Indiana, USA

CHIEF COMPLAINT AND HISTORY OF PRESENT ILLNESS

The patient is a 38-year-old medical salesperson who presented with progressive bilateral tibiofemoral joint line pain and activity-related swelling of his right knee. He had a history of medial and lateral meniscectomies performed at the time of anterior cruciate ligament (ACL) reconstruction approximately 8 years earlier. He had no functional instability and initially maintained an active lifestyle including running and basketball, until the gradual onset of medial greater than lateral joint line pain occurred. He has eliminated impact activities and changed to biking and swimming.

PHYSICAL EXAMINATION

Height, 5 ft, 8 in.; weight, 146 lb. Gait of right limb is stiff and mildly antalgic. Clinical alignment is varus with excellent muscle bulk and tone. The knee has a trace effusion. Range of motion is from 5 to 135 degrees of flexion. He has medial and lateral joint line tenderness without patellofemoral findings. His ligament examination is normal. His patellar tracking is normal.

RADIOGRAPHIC EVALUATION

Radiographs demonstrate prior ACL reconstruction with isolated joint space narrowing of the right knee medial compartment (Figure C38.1). Standing hip-to-ankle alignment films show 6 degrees of varus.

SURGICAL INTERVENTION

At staging arthroscopy, focal grade III to IV chondral lesions of the trochlea (1.5 cm by 2.3 cm) and medial femoral condyle (1.5 cm by 2.5 cm) were identified. Both menisci were essentially absent. The ACL graft was intact. In light of the varus alignment and medial pathology greater than lateral, the limb was treated at the time of staging arthroscopy with high tibial valgus-producing osteotomy using an opening-wedge hemicallotasis technique with an external fixator. The goal was to correct alignment such that the weight-bearing line would just enter the lateral compartment (Figure C38.2). Cartilage restoration was performed after the osteotomy had healed. Autologous chondrocyte implantation (ACI) was performed on the trochlea and medial femoral condyle defects

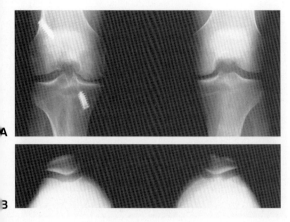

FIGURE C38.1. Preoperative 45-degree flexion weight-bearing posteroanterior **(A)** and Merchant **(B)** views demonstrate prior evidence of anterior cruciate ligament (ACL) reconstruction and minimal medial joint space narrowing.

(Figure C38.3). The medial and lateral meniscal transplants were performed through the same arthrotomy as the ACI, using tibial tubercle osteotomy for exposure and not for realignment (Figure C38.4).

Postoperatively, the patient was made nonweight bearing for 4 weeks and used immediate continuous passive motion during that time for 6 h/day. After 4 weeks, the patient was allowed to progress to weight bearing as tolerated with crutches. Once the patient lost his antalgic gait, the crutches were no longer used.

FOLLOW-UP

Postoperatively, his range of motion reached a plateau of 5 to 115 degrees of flexion. Ten months later, he developed recurrence of his medial pain and underwent arthroscopy. The ACI had largely incorporated, the lateral meniscal transplant had healed and appeared near normal (Figure C38.5), whereas the medial meniscus was torn at the posterior horn attachment. Debridement of the torn meniscus fragment and scar tissue allowed increased flexion to 125 degrees while maintaining extension. The area of incomplete filling by ACI was treated with microfracture. Thereafter, his pain was minimized to significantly less than his initial preoperative condition.

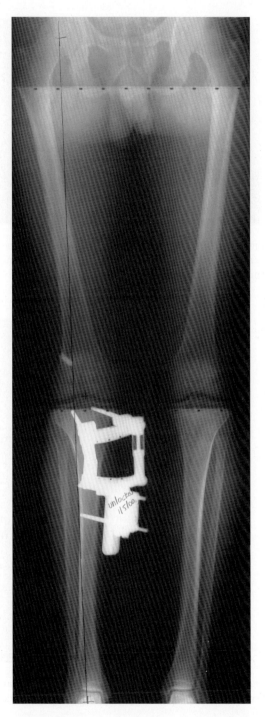

FIGURE C38.2. Postoperative radiograph with external fixator in place, and complete healing of the valgus-producing hemicallotasis high tibial osteotomy (HTO). Note that the weight-bearing line falls into the medial third of the lateral compartment.

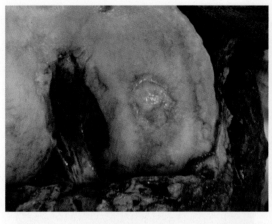

A   B

FIGURE C38.3. **(A)** Intraoperative views of the central trochlear and medial femoral condyle lesions (note intact ACL graft). **(B)** Autologous chondrocyte implantation (ACI) periosteal patch in place following preparation of the medial femoral condyle lesion.

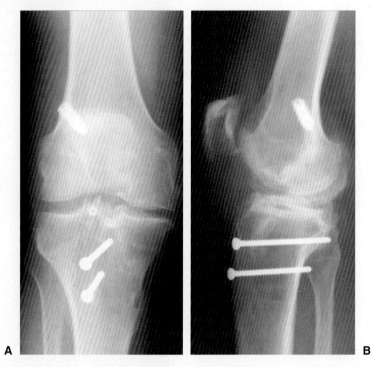

A   B

FIGURE C38.4. Postoperative anteroposterior **(A)** and lateral **(B)** films show evidence of medial and lateral bone bridge in slot meniscal transplants and fixation of the tibial tubercle.

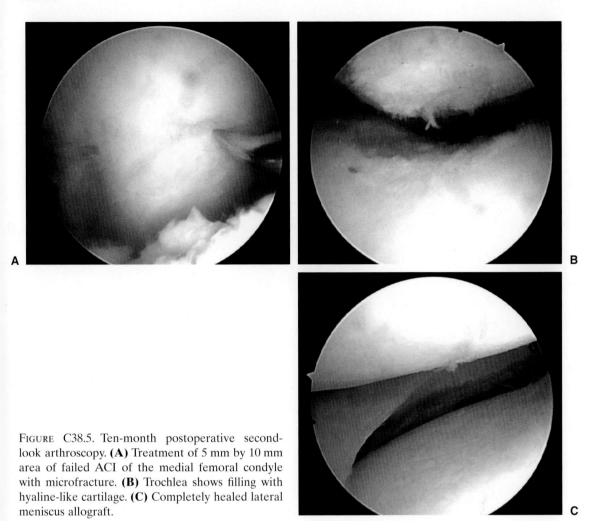

Figure C38.5. Ten-month postoperative second-look arthroscopy. **(A)** Treatment of 5 mm by 10 mm area of failed ACI of the medial femoral condyle with microfracture. **(B)** Trochlea shows filling with hyaline-like cartilage. **(C)** Completely healed lateral meniscus allograft.

DECISION-MAKING FACTORS

1. Young, active patient with progressive symptoms largely in the medial compartment, but also in the lateral compartment.
2. Staged osteotomy without efforts to overcorrect varus deformity due to bicompartmental nature of the patient's symptoms and disease.
3. Single-stage cartilage restoration procedure to treat both the chondral surfaces and meniscal deficiency such that each procedure provides relative protection against respective graft failure.
4. Minor complaints of anterior knee pain led to a decision to avoid a significant anteromedialization of the tibial tubercle with the tubercle osteotomy performed primarily for surgical exposure.
5. Indications for second look due to pain and motion loss led to management of incomplete ACI fill with microfracture and meniscal tearing with partial meniscectomy.

Index